The Crystal Healing Bible

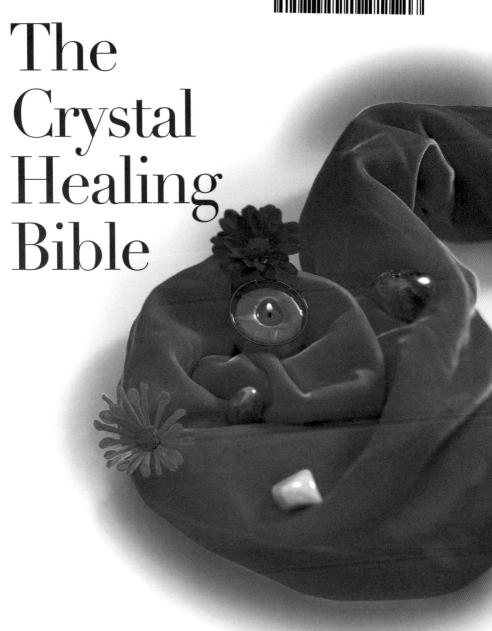

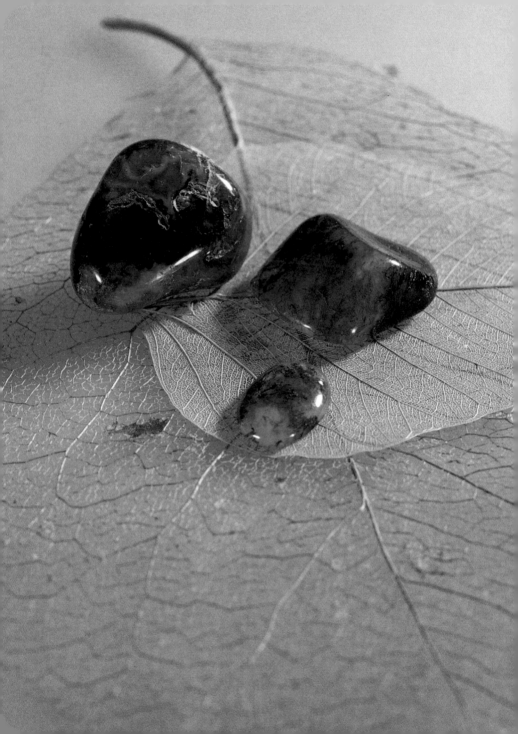

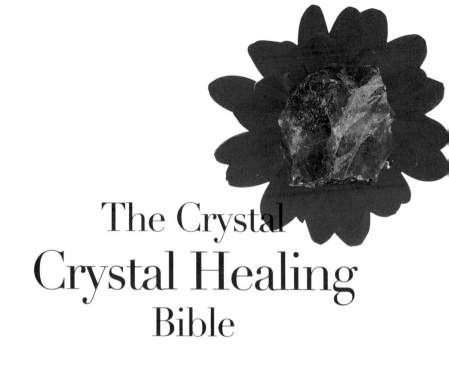

The Crystal
Crystal Healing
Bible

Practical divination techniques that
harness a million years of earth energy
to reveal your lives, loves and destiny

Sue Lilly

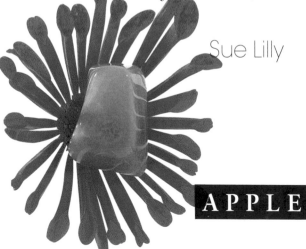

APPLE

A QUANTUM BOOK

This edition published in 2013 by
Apple Press
74-77 White Lion St
LondonN1 9PH

Copyright © 2012 Quantum Publishing
Ltd

ISBN: 978-1-84543-530-1

Produced by
Quantum Publishing Ltd
The Old Brewery
6 Blundell Street
London N7 9BH

QUMTECB

Assistant Editor: Jo Morley
Project Editor: Samantha Warrington
Managing Editor: Julie Brooke
Production Manager: Rohana Yusof
Publisher: Sarah Bloxham

Packaged by Gulmohur

Printed in China by Midas Printing
International Ltd.

Quantum would like to thank and acknowledge
the following for supplying the pictures
reproduced in this book:

(Key: l left, r right, c centre, t top, b bottom)

p16 The Art Archive; p17b Trip/c Gray; p27
Image Bank; p30/31 The Art Archive; p32 J-L
Charmet; p39 Image Bank; p40 Pictor; p42
Shutterstock; p45 The Art Archive; p64 The
Art Archive; p65 The Art Archive; p68t The Art
Archive, p68b Shutterstock; p71c Ruta Brown;
P78b Image Bank, p78t Pictor; p89 The Art
Archive; p91 Zzvet/Shutterstock; p95 Pictor;
p101bl Pictor; p104tr The Art Archive; p108
Shutterstock; p111c The Art Archive; p115
Shutterstock; p138 The Art Archive; p145
Thinkstock; p152 Pictor; p162t Pictor; p168t
The Art Archive; p168b Shutterstock; p169 The
Art Archive; p172 Shutterstock; p174c The Art
Archive; p177 The Art Archive; p188t The Art
Archive, p188b The Art Archive; p184tl Pictor
International; p185 The Art Archive; p194 The
Art Archive; p199 Pictor International; p204b
The Art Archive; p213 Image Bank

All other photographs and illustrations are the
copyright of Quantum Publishing Ltd

While every effort has been made to credit
contributors, Quantum would like to apologise
should there have been any omissions or errors.

The material in this book originally appeared in
The Crystal Decoder.

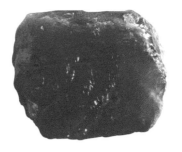

Contents

Foreword 6

Introduction **8**
Where do Crystals Come from? 10
Crystal Energy 14
Healing Powers of Crystals 16
Sitting with a Crystal 18

Divination **20**
Traditions and Techniques 22
The Principles of Crystal Reading 26
Choosing Your Personal Stone 30
Setting the Scene 36
Balancing Your Mind 38
Methods of Crystal Reading 40
Pendulum Dowsing 48
Casting the Crystals 50
Interpreting the Crystals 52
Interpreting the Compass Board 54
Interpreting the Astrological Board 57

The Crystal Directory **60**

Crystal Magic **214**

Index 224

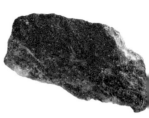

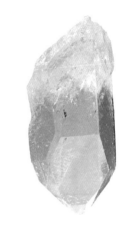

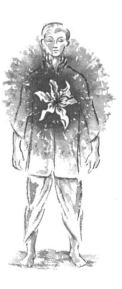

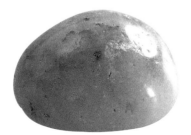

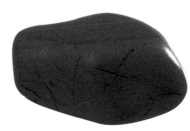

Foreword

There are many books available on the subject of divination, yet only a small number have been written exclusively on the subject of crystals. Crystals, along with all other types of stones, have been used for healing and divination purposes since time immemorial. In ancient times, shamans and tribal healers used stones as tools for healing the sick and for divinatory work; today, alternative healers and diviners continue this age-old tradition.

Like all natural objects, crystals are magical tools which we can use to effect change and achieve harmonisation. They have the power to help us along our individual paths through the maze of life by expanding our consciousness, calming our stresses, and infusing us with healing energies. Just as importantly, as natural tools, they can help us reconnect to the Earth and the universe in the midst of this technological age.

Written by an exceptionally proficient tutor and consultant, this book provides a wealth of knowledge on many aspects of the fascinating subject of crystals. In explaining some of the most important divination systems centred around crystals, and in detailing the healing powers commonly attributed to forty-five of the most powerful crystals, this book will no doubt prove an invaluable resource for those who seek to empower themselves and to improve their lives. I am sure that this book will be treasured and appreciated by both crystal novices and experts alike, whether as an introduction to the world of crystals, as a source of further insight for those already in tune to the powers of crystals, or simply as a way to enhance one's enjoyment of crystals.

Thank you, Sue, for allowing us to share in your wisdom.

Berenice Watt, president of the British Astrological and Psychic Society (1994–99)

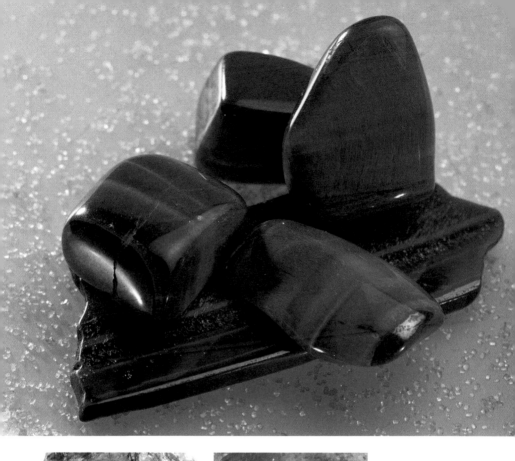

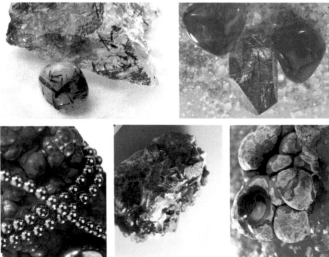

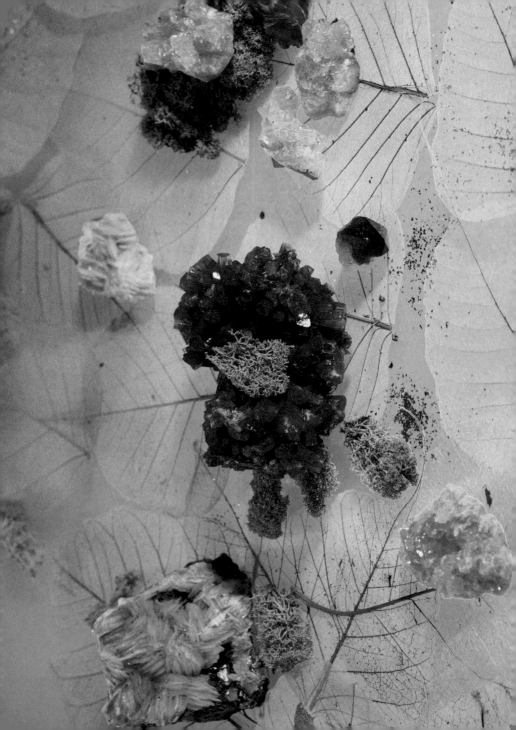

Introduction

The mineral kingdom and the crystals it contains are the foundation of all physical matter and of life itself. Crystals are the most orderly, most stable forms of matter in the entire universe. Their beauty, striking colours, and forms have always attracted attention, and yet their value goes far beyond surface appearance.

Where Do Crystals Come From?

Crystals are all around us, from sand and pebbles on the beach to the finely polished slabs decorating the façades of government buildings. For centuries precious stones have been collected from riverbanks and dug out of the sides of hills and mountains wherever erosion has uncovered the sparkling caves and crevices. We see crystals at the end of a long process. It often takes millions of years before they emerge into the light of day.

Sliding layers

The planet Earth appears firm, solid, and stable, but in reality the solid rock continents upon which we live are only the thinnest of skins covering a turbulent, swirling, and dynamic interior. The planet's own rotation, its orbit around the sun, and the influence of the moon and other planets all create huge gravitational forces within the massive volumes of rock in the Earth's mantle. These layers slide over each other in a continuous movement.

Crystallisation

Stresses can fracture the brittle layers of rock in the Earth's crust. This is where crystals can form, as heated gases and liquids under huge pressures force their way upward toward the surface, together with hot molten rock known as magma. These solutions are saturated with different elements and compounds – water, oxygen, sodium, gold, and iron, for example – that have dissolved from the deep layers within the mantle. As they pass through cooler, less active layers of rock, these elements fall out of solution and begin to crystallise in cavities and crevices. Depending on the mix of elements and environmental conditions, different minerals will form. The

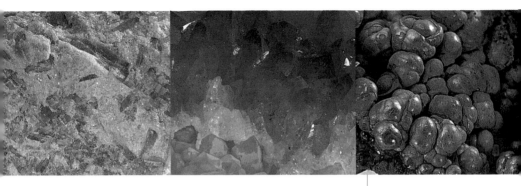

original amount of each raw material will determine the size of the crystals and the extent of each deposit.

Although not all crystals form in these volcanic, or igneous, conditions, many of the most precious gemstones do form in this way. These are usually the harder stones, such as garnet, ruby, and diamond. The borders of igneous activity around volcanoes are known as rich areas of mineralization.

Altered conditions

As the Earth's crust is in a state of continuous – albeit slow – change, conditions can alter, allowing successive waves of crystallisation. Where rocks and minerals are changed into completely new structures and compositions by this successive crystallisation, the conditions are called metamorphic. Metamorphic rocks and their attendant crystals occur in areas of great heat and pressure, often where rocks are buried, folded, and compressed by the Earth's movements.

As soon as they are exposed to water, wind, and ice, all rocks will begin to erode. Tons of rock particles are washed down rivers every day, settling in mud banks or being carried to the sea. Over millions of years, these deposits build up to an enormous thickness. Their weight, combined with that of the water above them, compresses the layers together to form another type of rock: sedimentary. Sedimentary rock tends to be more delicate than crystals that have formed under volcanic or metamorphic conditions.

Above Rubellite in lepidolite forms in a pegmatite; citrine results from superheated solution; hematite is created when certain minerals are broken down by water.

11

Crystal characteristics

No matter where they form, all crystals have the same basic characteristics. Furthermore, any mineral or chemical compound can form crystals, given the right conditions, and every mineral's crystals will have the same arrangement of constituent atoms throughout, which will be reflected in the geometric shapes visible in its faces, sides, and angles.

Crystal sizes range from extremely small to several feet long. Rose quartz crystals, for example, are microscopically small (or microcrystalline); they take what is called massive form, where small crystals intergrow. With this type of crystal, no regular geometrical shapes can be seen. Many members of the quartz family are microcrystalline, usually because they form from solution in relatively low temperatures, and thus do not have the energy to form large crystals.

Crystal formation

Crystals will form wherever they have space to grow and, wherever possible, each will grow away from other crystals nearby. Seed crystals will begin to form on the surrounding bedrock or matrix. Very often, a microcrystalline layer appears first, before larger, separate crystals eventually emerge.

Where hot magma remains at a constant temperature for a long time, very large crystals can grow. This formation is known as a pegmatite. Many different sorts of minerals may crystallise along the length of a pegmatite, and some may even intergrow. Where there is a hollow space that is an enclosed bubble originally created by gas or liquid, mineral-rich solutions can seep in and crystallise. Depending on the conditions, either large crystals or layers of small microcrystalline crystals can grow here. These geodes, as they are called, are the main sources of amethyst, as well as other banded agates.

Colour variation

The variations in crystal colour derive from minuscule amounts of different elements that create impurities within the crystal structure. In most instances, colour is created when these small impurities alter

Facing Page Bottom Left Veins rich in minerals such as gold and iron are formed when hot magma packed with minerals seeps upward through cracks.

Facing Page Bottom Right Many crystals form when water is heated by magma underground and becomes enriched with minerals.

the internal structure of the crystal so that light rays are bent toward one or the other end of the spectrum. In fact, to the confusion of the novice, most crystals can form in a wide range of different colours; this confusion is amplified when the same mineral is given a different name, depending on its colour.

Learning to recognise the habit of a mineral – the common ways in which the crystals form together, their range of shapes and colours, and how they look both in a natural form and as a polished gemstone – is all part of familiarising oneself with the energy of crystals.

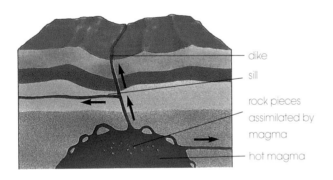

dike

sill

rock pieces assimilated by magma

hot magma

Left Magma can give birth to many kinds of crystals as it cools and interacts with the native rock in many ways, each subtly changing the magma's chemical composition.

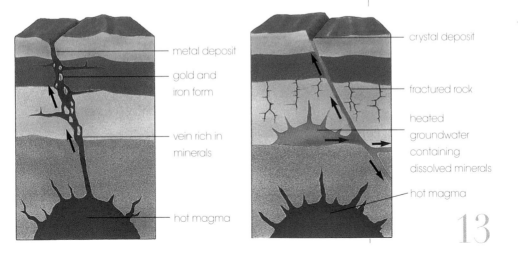

metal deposit

gold and iron form

vein rich in minerals

hot magma

crystal deposit

fractured rock

heated groundwater containing dissolved minerals

hot magma

13

Crystal Energy

Humankind has been using crystals and minerals for millennia, and they continue to be integral to our lives today. Not only do we find them in complex machinery, engines, gauges, satellites, and space shuttles, but they are also used for making dyes, paints, and medicines. They even form part of our diets, as salt.

Structure and form

The special qualities of crystals – that which makes them visually fascinating and technologically useful – arise from the way in which they are formed, deep within the planet. When crystals begin to grow out of superheated solutions, their constituent atoms are free to combine, and do so in the most stable arrangements possible. Each crystal quickly builds up a characteristic three-dimensional pattern of atoms called a crystal lattice, which repeats itself throughout the entire crystal structure until there are no more free atoms available. As the availability of raw materials declines, the lattice begins to reduce in size. The regular prismatic sides form the points and terminations of the crystals.

Crystals are the most stable forms of matter in the universe. Having grown into their ideal solid forms, they possess energy that derives from their essential orderliness. Comfortable in their atomic arrangement, crystals are excellent at resisting external energies. For example, when their structure is compressed, many crystals will emit the resultant excess energy as light or an electric charge. Conversely, if an electric current is fed into a crystal, the crystal will respond by expanding slightly to accommodate the extra energy input.

An alternating current will create a regular pulsing in the structure of a quartz crystal. This energy has been used to replace the clockwork mechanism of watches, although today, the quartz used is usually artificial.

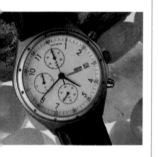

Above Many everyday items, including watches and radios, depend upon quartz crystals to function efficiently.

Rays of light

A crystal's lattice structure determines how light will pass through, or between, its atoms. Some minerals – quartz, for example – allow rays of light to pass through almost unchanged, although the light does slow down fractionally. Other crystals split light into different beams, creating a polarising effect. Tourmaline, for example, shows different colours, depending on the angle from which it is viewed. Calcite bounces light back off its surfaces to create a double image, called double refraction.

The behaviour of light when it encounters a crystal lattice often produces the crystal colours we see. With transparent or translucent crystals, the resulting intense colouration introduces a very particular energy into the environment – whether into a room or into a person's energy field or aura. No other natural material can focus and concentrate the frequencies of light in such a consistent way.

Natural energy resonators

The behaviour of crystals can be explained in terms of physics – particularly the area of solid-state physics that deals with energies at subatomic levels – but it is unwise to make direct comparisons to their uses in the contexts of healing and spiritual growth. Only some very tentative suggestions can be offered.

Crystals are the most orderly and the simplest solid matter in the universe. Orderliness and simplicity in any form always brings chaotic energies into a greater state of order; this phenomenon is known as the principle of resonance. Crystals can be thought of as natural energy resonators. Some crystal healers believe that the dynamism of the body recognises the crystal's orderly simplicity. According to this view, the crystal acts as a template against which the body's self-regulatory functions can perform more efficiently, encouraging a move toward health or clarity of perception. Crystals can be very effective tools for releasing emotional stress and restoring calm to anxious individuals.

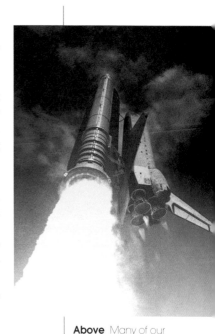

Above Many of our most impressive technological developments are dependent upon crystal and mineral components in order to function properly.

15

Healing Powers of Crystals

Quartz, or rock crystal, has long played an important role in many cultures as a tool for healing and divination. Today the popular use of jewellery and birthstone amulets continues our centuries-old relationship with the subtle energies of crystals and gemstones.

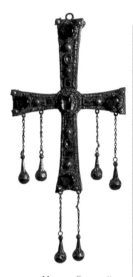

Above Encrusting symbolic religious items with gemstones enhanced their magical power as well as their appearance.

Among the native tribes of North America, quartz crystals were traditionally used to forecast the outcome of a hunt or battle. The stone would either be gazed into, like a crystal ball, in search of indications of success or failure; or it would be held in sunlight, and the reflected light was interpreted in accordance with where it fell.

In some traditions, healers would use quartz to examine a patient. The areas of disease, once located, were removed by rubbing the crystal over the body to draw out the imbalances. In such cases, it was the spirit of the stone that became the means of healing, and it was the spirit who was propitiated before, and thanked after, the healing session.

Ceremonies and rituals

In ancient times, certain stones clearly held important places in ceremony and everyday ritual. Old Indian texts describe the origin of gemstones and define their beneficial powers. Coral, carnelian, turquoise, abalone shell, and obsidian were used throughout the Americas as protective amulets. In Central America, turquoise and jade were the favoured materials to offer as ritual ornaments to the temple gods.

In Indonesia and Australasia, quartz is the primary stone used for divination and conversing with the spirits. The Aborigines of Australia use quartz as a symbolic means of initiation into healing and sorcery. Across the Pacific islands, quartz is regarded as belonging to the realm of the spirits, ancestors, and creator gods.

16

Healing methods

There is little evidence that crystals are used as healing tools today in the same ways in which they were used in ancient times. Contemporary reports from Tibet and Peru suggest that some healers do use stones to place on and around the body to remove illness, but these are more often ordinary-looking rocks and pebbles than mineral crystals.

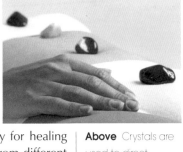

Above Crystals are used to direct spiritual healing energy from the healer into the patient.

The placing of stones on and around the body for healing purposes seems to be an amalgamation of ideas from different traditions. Knowledge from India and Tibet on the subtle anatomy of the human body – particularly the seven main chakra centres – has been combined with colour therapy theories that connect parts of the body with each of the colours of the rainbow spectrum. This interpretation seems to have occurred as a result of translations done in the early nineteenth and twentieth centuries of Indian texts by the Theosophical Society.

In another method of healing, crystals are used to direct or amplify healing energy that flows from the healer into the patient's auric field – a sort of supercharged spiritual healing. Today, crystal healing is looked upon by many as one of the more bizarre manifestations of the alternative scene. Its reputation has not been helped by the rather fabulous – and unsubstantiated – claims by some of its more outspoken promoters, such as the declaration that crystals were used in Atlantis.

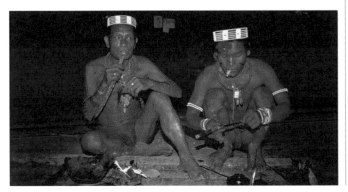

Left Healers and shamans use a wide variety of tools to help them communicate with the spirits. In some traditions, stones or crystals are used.

17

Sitting with a Crystal

Each time you acquire a new crystal, take time to explore how it changes your self-awareness. The more familiar you become with each stone's energy, the greater your insights relating to its uses and meanings will be.

Repeat this below routine as often as you like. It is a good idea to take notes during or immediately after the procedure, before any details are forgotten.

1. Start by settling yourself into a comfortable seat. Place the stone you wish to explore in front of you at a height from which you can gaze at it without straining your eyes.

2. Begin by closing your eyes, taking a couple of deep breaths, then gently turning your attention to how you are feeling.

3. First, tune in to your body and think about how it feels. Are there areas of tension or discomfort, or is there some other sensation?

4. Next, direct your attention to your emotional state and your thoughts Are you experiencing a pervading mood? Is your mind active or quiet? Are you focusing on certain issues?

5. Once you have explored your own energy state, turn your attention toward the stone. To begin with, simply gaze at the crystal in front of you for a minute or two.

6. Close your eyes and scan your body, mind, and emotions once more, to see if you can notice any differences, however slight.

7. Next, pick up the stone and examine it closely from all angles.

8. Hold the stone between your hands and close your eyes again. Note any changes that occur in the next few minutes.

You can also learn how a stone is affecting you by carrying or wearing it for a couple of days and then leaving it behind for another couple of days. Experimenting in this way, you will gather more useful knowledge about your stones than you could ever glean from reading about them. At the same time, you will be developing your sensitivity to crystals.

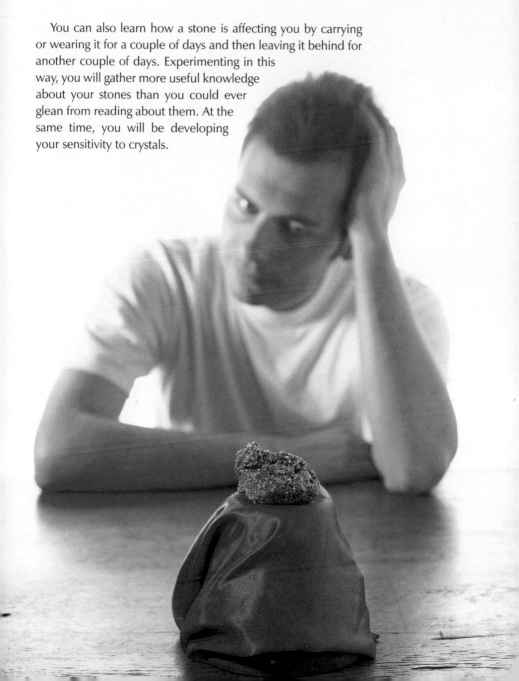

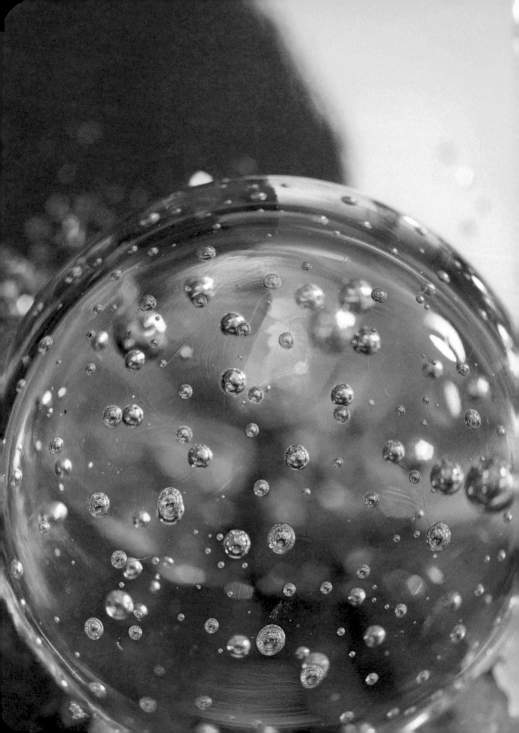

Divination

Divination is a way of clearing a straight,
clear path to the future by paying attention
to details and events so small as to escape
ordinary notice, or to be thought irrelevant. In
the world of divination, we learn that nothing
is unimportant because all things are, at some
level, interconnected. The diviner reads the
world for signs of underlying energies that will
shape future events or lives.

Traditions and Techniques

Diviners are, by and large, practical people who, once their skills have been honed, are able to use whatever materials are at hand, whether it be bones, stones, dice, or a candle flame. Effective methods are passed down through tradition, but the most important tool of the trade is the mind of the diviner. All the casting techniques, props, and prayers are useless unless they help the diviner achieve the state of awareness that is necessary in order to interpret the signs correctly.

Ancient methods

Because historical and archaeological records regarding ancient crystal casting are incomplete, it can be difficult to correctly interpret the past uses to which various artefacts have been put. For example, a string of beads may have been worn as a decorative necklace, but the owner may also have used the beads to divine, as some cultures did. In the ancient Tibetan system of divination, called Mo, after the questioner asks the question and repeats the necessary mantras, beads are counted back in groups, leaving a maximum of six beads. Each number of remaining beads from one to six has a meaning ranging from "excellent" to "terrible," and thus the questioner is informed as to the likely outcome of the venture.

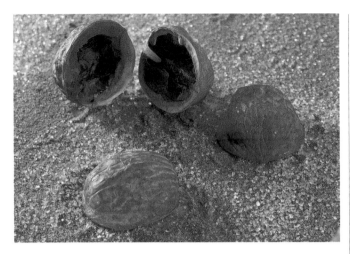

Crystals have long been used as a way of communicating with the spirit worlds and, through scrying (the act of gazing into a crystal ball), of looking into a window to the future. Natural crystals, polished spheres, and smooth mirrored surfaces have all been used in divination. Ordinary stones have likewise played a major role in divination techniques, especially the casting technique.

Playing with time

Humanity's confusion – the very reason why there is a need for oracles at all – is caused by our experience of time as a linear flow, from past, to present, to future. We exist in the present and can remember the past, but the future can only be guessed at. We always seem to be heading into the unknown. And yet, in other states of awareness, time is more elastic and flexible. In dreams, for example, the past, present, and future interact within their own form of logic, echoing the essential secret of divination: it is possible to free the mind from the limits of the ordinary universe. In other words, the mind, not being a physical entity, is not constrained by the laws of time and space.

Our experience of time is very much tied to our metabolic rate – the speed of our lives. For a creature with a rapid

23

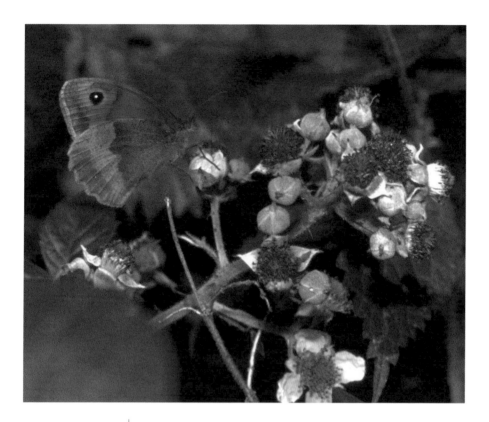

metabolism, such as a rabbit, an hour might seem to stretch out forever, because so much activity is crowded into that time. For a being with a slower metabolism – a tree, for example – a year might seem equivalent to our notion of a single day.

Crystals are the most stable matter in the universe. Once created, if left alone, they can remain in the same form for millenia. What experience of time do crystals have? Probably one of seeing the entire history of humankind flash by in a minute! In this way, crystals are quite removed from the flow of time. They are also free from the constraint of space: although each crystal is unique in form, its internal structure is constant in all samples of that mineral, wherever they are found across the universe.

Casting techniques

Whereas scrying (meaning "seeing") opens the clairvoyant faculties of the diviner's mind, casting techniques follow predetermined rules of interpretation.

Casting divination techniques can take three main forms. In the simplest methods, the cast items have no significance or individual meaning. Very often there is a simple heads-or-tails approach, with shells or nuts landing on one side or the other. The various combinations provide the answer to the question at hand. The African system of Ifa, the Chinese I Ching, and some types of geomancy fall within this category.

In the second type of casting, each object has a specific and identifiable set of meanings. The way that each item falls in relation to the others creates a picture of which energies are involved with each other, suggesting the likely outcome. The Germanic runes, and possibly the Celtic systems of Coelbran, used this method. Similarly, the bone oracles of South Africa employ a series of different items, the precise fall of which indicates a set outcome.

The third method of casting involves a set grid or map onto which the objects are cast. Each segment of the grid or map is ascribed a definite meaning. The cast object's fall can be interpreted either from where it lands or, in more complex systems, from the specific meaning given to each object, which is then modified by where it falls in the casting area. In the art of geomancy (literally "divination by earth"), for example, not only is the dispersion of the stones or the number of marks made important – the places where they fall or occur upon a set of predetermined grids is the key element. The use of a specially designed board for casting – the Compass or Astrological designs, for example (see pages 40–42 and 43–45) – allows for a precise interpretation for each placement.

Facing page and Below For creatures of the animal kingdom, the flow of real time is experienced as body time. Small animals such as butterflies have rapid metabolic rates, and thus shorter life spans, whereas large animals such as elephants have slower metabolic rates, resulting in longer life spans.

The Principles of Crystal Reading

The principles of all oracles and divination are derived from the ancient world view of our tribal ancestors, who observed that all things and all events were inextricably tied together in a complex web of interaction. To most people at most times, this web is impossible to comprehend. But at certain special times – and for people with the ability to step between worlds and glimpse the web – it is possible to see how some strands interconnect.

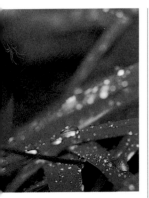

Above In many cultures, the spider represents the creator goddess, weaving the world from her body.

Spirits and the unconscious

In the primeval world view, everything has a spirit, and everything is alive. What most of us perceive to be going on in the world is often only an outer, visible indication of a reality that exists within a greater spiritual world. Therefore, if one can learn to pose the right questions to the spirits in the correct manner, why should they not answer?

In his study of the unconscious, the psychologist Carl Jung explored the idea of a universal web, as well as the occurrence of simultaneous significant events with no apparent causal link. Modern research has also highlighted aspects of the universal web theory in the phenomenon known as the "hundredth monkey." This phenomenon occurs when a threshold number of individuals within a species – one in one hundred – has learned something new. Once this proportion of individuals has learned the new information, it appears that the information transfers to the entire population virtually instantly. Similarly, physics and mathematics have uncovered the chaos theory, which shows that seemingly random events reveal endless complexities of orderly patterning.

The inner mind, otherwise known as the unconscious – or that part of ourselves not usually noticed in the everyday rambling thought processes of conscious awareness – is able to access some of this underlying pattern-making at an intuitive level. However, linear thought cannot exist at this level of awareness, so messages must be sent in another form. Our unconscious mind speaks to our conscious mind by making us notice seemingly insignificant events, or by making connections, associations or symbolic links. These connections, associations, or links can reveal underlying patterns that may determine future events which will materialise into our conscious reality.

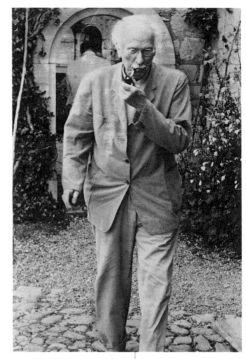

Learning to divine

Learning to divine is all about learning how to dip into nonverbal layers of awareness. A random casting of stones has no inherent meaning, so the conscious mind is left directionless. But the intuitive mind connects the question asked to the fall of stones, and can recognise significant patterns. It is then the job of the diviner to bring that information to the surface in a useful way.

Above Carl Jung was an important influence on the development of contemporary interest in divination and the powers of the mind.

In any reading, there will always be more than one possible interpretation. The beginner always frets about which one is right, but the answer to these worries is to let the meanings float up to your mind and go with whatever association comes up first. No one else can interpret your oracle for you because it is your mind that is the oracle – the stones, the board, and all other paraphernalia are simply tools that you can use to help you focus. The answers are within your mind, not in any divination object you are using. With practice, you will begin to recognise the feel of a correct interpretation.

Giving a successful reading

The role of the diviner is to help clear up the confusion of the questioner – the person who has asked for the reading. If the questioner's confusion is lessened by the end of the session, then the session can be deemed a success, no matter how accurate the diviner feels the reading has been.

It is very important that in the reading process both the diviner and the questioner are clear that this is not a test of clairvoyance, spiritual powers, or any other supernatural skill. Divining is not mind reading. The questioner should be open and willing to receive advice, and should be willing to provide whatever information the diviner needs to clarify the answer given by the cast.

The diviner also needs to take care how the interpretation is given. If you are the diviner, you must always remember that nothing is free from change. Even taking advice from a divination technique can significantly alter the likely outcome of any event. Avoid at all costs the curse of prophecy. Many mediocre and poor diviners insist that what they see will come to pass exactly as they see it. Where is free will in this interpretation? Where, indeed, are compassion and understanding? The diviner is there to advise, not to foretell. Foretelling is no different from cursing, because it sets up a strong tendency in the minds of both the diviner and questioner to work toward that outcome. Further, foretelling inextricably links the future actions of the questioner with the diviner, since the diviner has become a significant cause of those actions.

Divining should be a process of exploring possibilities. Clarity is the desired outcome, and both diviner and questioner should be working together toward this end. The web has infinite threads, along which anyone may travel. But a web is also full of holes that one can fall through. It is the job of the diviner to focus on the threads that may be of use in traversing the unknown voids of existence – not to distract the questioner with silly or trite observations.

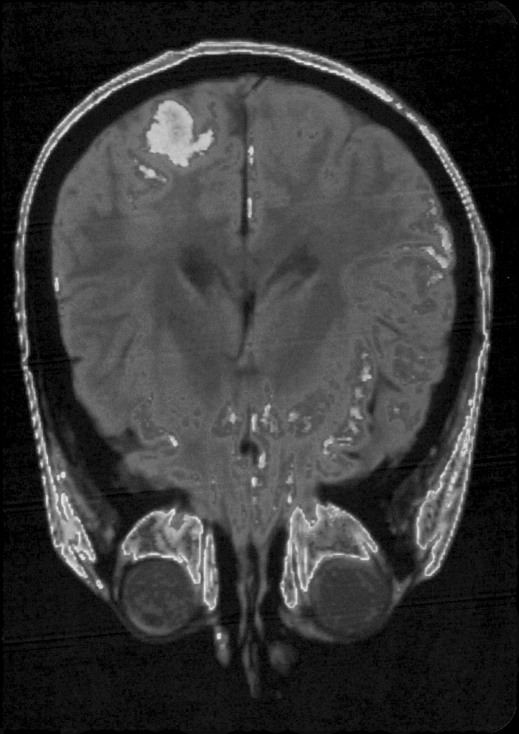

Choosing Your Personal Stone

There are several guidelines that the questioner can follow when choosing a personal stone. The questioner can choose his or her own stone if doing the reading for him- or herself, or if the reading is done on his or her behalf by another. If the questioner is absent during the reading, the diviner can choose a stone on his or her behalf. The choice of a personal stone can be made in a number of ways. There are Eastern and Western systems in place that can be used as guidelines; or, one may choose not to follow any existing system, opting instead for an intuitive approach. All three methods are outlined in the next few pages.

Above Since ancient times, the zodiac signs have been associated with certain parts of the human body. In this way, each person becomes a tiny version of the universe.

Eastern systems

In the early Ayurvedic and Tantric texts, certain gems were related to specific parts of the human body. Wearing these gems was believed to help heal the relevant body parts, and to support an individual's progress in life. There were nine stones related to the planets and the nodes of the moon (points in space related to the movement of the moon and the apparent movement of the sun), with four extra stones related solely to the body.

The chart on the lower half of the facing page shows the planets and their corresponding body parts and crystals, plus acceptable substitutes. You can use it as a guideline when choosing your own personal stone, or if choosing a stone for a questioner for whom you will be divining. This system of choosing a stone is particularly useful if the questioner is having problems with any of the body parts named. The choice of the relevant crystal will help alleviate the illness.

Gem	Main signs	Secondary signs	Signs that should avoid this gem
ruby	Leo	Aries	Libra, Aquarius
pearl	Cancer	Taurus	Scorpio, Capricorn
coral	Aries, Scorpio	Capricorn	Cancer, Libra, Taurus
emerald	Gemini, Virgo	Virgo	Pisces, Sagittarius
topaz	Sagittarius, Pisces	Cancer	Capricorn, Gemini, Virgo
diamond	Libra, Taurus	Pisces	Virgo, Aries, Scorpio
blue sapphire	Aquarius, Capricorn	Libra	Aries, Leo, Cancer
amethyst	Taurus		Scorpio
cat's-eye	Scorpio		Taurus

Planet	Body part	Original crystals	Acceptable substitutes
Sun	blood	ruby	rose quartz, garnet, spinel, zircon
Moon	teeth	pearl	moon-stone, quartz
Mercury	bile	emerald	aquamarine, peridot, jade, green tourmaline
Venus	bones	diamond	white stones
Mars	intestines	coral	carnelian, red jasper
Jupiter	skin	yellow sapphire	topaz, citrine
Saturn	eyes	blue sapphire	amethyst, lapis lazuli
Rahu (north node)	semen/ ovum	hessonite garnet	
Ketu (south node)	sound	cat's-eye (chrysoberyl)	
	nails	tourmaline	
	sight/liver	lapis lazuli	
	whole body	agate	
	spleen	quartz	

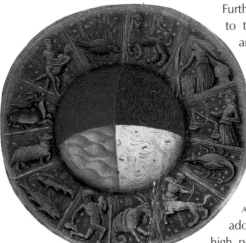

Further Ayurvedic correspondences were linked to the signs of the zodiac. Certain gemstones are strongly connected to certain signs, with other secondary signs connected – albeit less strongly – to the gemstones as well. In this system, there are specific gems that should be avoided for each sign. The chart on the upper half of the previous page shows how to choose a stone using this system.

Western systems

In the West, as early as the fifth century AD, writers have linked the twelve stones that adorned the breastplate of the biblical Hebrew high priest to the twelve signs of the zodiac, and later to the twelve months of the year. But it was not until 1912, at a meeting of the U.S. National Association of Jewelers, in Kansas, that a general consensus was reached as to an agreed pairing of birthstones and crystals with months of the year and signs of the zodiac. The lists below this page and the opposite page are widely held to be the definitive guides.

Above The present-day zodiac wheel, with its animals and figures, derives from the ancient Greeks.

Month	Birthstone
January	garnet
February	amethyst
March	bloodstone, aquamarine, jasper
April	diamond, sapphire
May	emerald, agate
June	pearl, moonstone, emerald
July	ruby, onyx
August	peridot, carnelian
September	sapphire
October	opal, tourmaline, aquamarine
November	topaz
December	turquoise, lapis lazuli, ruby

Other ways to choose your personal stone

Following Eastern or Western guidelines is just one way of choosing your personal stone. There are currently a great many crystals that are easily available and, year by year, even more are finding their ways into our lives. You may thus wish to choose your personal stone by sight, instinct, after having undertaken research, or even randomly.

Preference

Arguably, the best reason for choosing a particular personal stone is because you like it. When we desire something, it is because seeing it creates changes in our internal chemistry, helping us to feel good. Having a particular preference gives each of us a means of showing our individuality. It is true that preferences change, and this could be an argument against choice as a way of determining a personal stone. However, since we are constantly changing and growing, it also makes sense that our personal stone should change along with us. Some people find their instinctive choice does in fact stay with them for the whole of their lives. Often such a stone reflects key factors of the individual's personality and behavioural patterns.

Star sign	Dates	Crystals
Aries	March 20–April 21	diamond, bloodstone, aquamarine, emerald
Taurus	April 21–May 22	emerald, diamond
Gemini	May 22–June 22	pearl, moonstone, agate, emerald
Cancer	June 22–July 23	ruby, emerald
Leo	July 23–August 24	ruby, peridot, turquoise
Virgo	August 24–September 23	opal, tourmaline, peridot
Libra	September 23–October 23	opal, tourmaline, sapphire, topaz
Scorpio	October 23–November 23	topaz, opal, aquamarine
Sagittarius	November 23–December 22	turquoise, garnet, topaz
Capricorn	December 22–January 21	garnet, turquoise
Aquarius	January 21–February 19	amethyst, garnet, ruby, diamond, jade
Pisces	February 19–March 20	aquamarine, bloodstone, amethyst, jasper

Colour

Colour is one of the greatest attractions of crystals. Our instinctive reaction to colour is so automatic that it takes vigilance to detect the subtle changes when we encounter different colours. Some reactions tend to be emotional, ranging from "Delicious! I could eat it!" to "Get that out of my sight!" – and all points in between. The following method can help you instinctively choose a personal stone.

1. Have before you a selection of stones.
2. Close your eyes and allow your breathing to settle.
3. Have the intention that, when you open your eyes, you will be drawn to a crystal that is appropriate for your personal stone.
4. Open your eyes and pay attention to where they come to rest.
5. The crystal upon which your gaze has fallen can become your personal stone.

This method can be used to select personal stones for each reading. It can also be used to find stones that will help you over longer periods of time, or for particular purposes. Just make sure that you have a clear intention in your mind before you select your stone.

Below Choosing a personal stone by sight is both the easiest and most intuitive method, as we typically feel drawn to that stone which immediately attracts our attention.

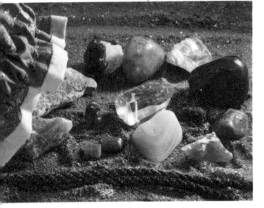

Reading about the qualities of stones

Some people may prefer a more logical approach when choosing a personal stone. Over the last thirty or forty years, many books have been written detailing the qualities and possible uses of crystals. Reading about crystals in these sources is a good way to get an overall assessment of how they are commonly perceived by those who have studied their powers and properties.

If this method is chosen, it is a good idea to look at as many sources as possible. Some crystals will seem to match your personality characteristics quite closely; these would make useful personal stones. Another approach is to select your stone according to the qualities that you wish to develop within yourself. If you wish to improve your patience, for example, a dark blue stone would be your best choice, and you would be well advised to steer clear of red, orange, and yellow stones. See pages 60–213 to find out the characteristics associated with each of the stones featured in this book.

Random selection

A random choice of a personal stone can be ideal for doing readings, or even just for choosing a stone for the day. The following two methods work particularly well.

Method one

1. Place all your stones inside a cloth bag.
2. Relax and slow your breathing down.
3. Have in your mind a clear intention to find a personal stone for the reading or for that day.
4. Dip your hand into the bag and pull out one stone.
5. If you like, you can look up the stone you have chosen; it may provide you with relevant advice or guidance.

Method two

1. Cut or tear as many small pieces of paper as you have stones.
2. Write your name on one piece of paper, shuffle all the papers and then lay them face down.
3. Place a stone on top of each of the pieces of paper.
4. When every piece of paper has a stone on it, turn each paper over until you find the one with your name under it. This can be your personal crystal, or your crystal for the day. Look up the meaning associated with your chosen crystal for additional insight.

Setting the Scene

Before you do any work with your crystals, they need to be cleansed to ensure that they are free of all outside influences and energies. Most hard crystals (from 3 or above on the Mohs scale, which indicates the relative hardness of minerals) can be safely washed in slightly soapy water. Softer crystals may become damaged by washing, and so other methods of cleansing will be necessary. Below are a variety of alternatives to cleansing.

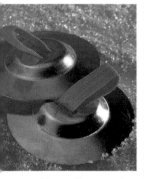

Above The use of hand cymbals is an easy way to cleanse your crystals.

Sound

Another easy cleansing method involves the use of bells, hand cymbals, or singing bowls. Sound of a fine quality and piercing resonance will help the crystals release any negative energy. If placing crystals in a singing bowl, put a small piece of fabric in the bottom to help stop them from rattling together.

Incense

Incense is an easy and effective cleansing method. Each stone can be passed through the incense smoke several times. Traditional purifying incenses, such as sandalwood, frankincense, and pine, are popular, as are the white sage and cedars traditionally used by Native Americans to cleanse their ritual spaces. Another option is to tie dried lavender stalks together and burn them, as they give off a pleasing aromatic smoke. The burning of bay leaves makes a pungent cleansing smoke.

Salt

It is inadvisable to use salted water for cleansing, as the salt crystals lodge in the crevices of the crystals being cleansed and can dull some surfaces. Dry sea salt can, however, be used; simply pile it onto the crystals to be cleansed and leave for 24 hours. (Don't use the salt for cooking afterwards!)

Preparing the physical space

The space in which the reading will take place can be as simple or as ornate as you wish. Following a specific routine can be very useful in setting the scene. Here are some suggestions for you to consider:

1. Whether you do your readings in bright or dim surroundings is really a personal decision. When we are relaxed and secure, the intuitive faculties work best, so decide what you feel most comfortable with.
2. You may want to have a small lamp or lighted candle nearby.
3. Choose a cloth to go under the board. The colour of the cloth is up to you. Black is the colour most often connected with any sort of reading, although deep reds and golds can be more welcoming.
4. Small objects such as flowers, talismans, or spiritual images may also feel appropriate in the space.
5. If you will be divining using a divinatory board, you may want to make a decision about which direction the board will face when you read. This consideration is particularly apt for the Compass board (see page 41). For example, you may prefer to align the North position on the board to the north of the room. You may also have a preference as to where you will sit.
6. Think about how your crystals are going to be presented – in an open display, or in a closed bag or box.

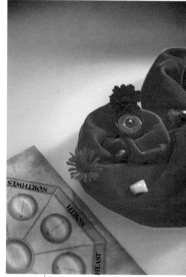

Above Choose items that will help you relax your mind and create a sacred space for your reading. As sacred space is naturally removed from our normal experience of time and space, it helps to facilitate the divination process.

Final considerations

When the scene is set, light some incense and leave the room to prepare yourself. Make sure that you will not be disturbed by the telephone or doorbell, or by any children or pets. Light the candle or switch on the lamp as you sit down to do the reading.

When the reading is finished, snuff out the candle or switch off the lamp. Clear away all your tools, then cleanse your crystals. Light some more incense if you wish, then leave the room empty for a while.

Balancing Your Mind

Preparation by the diviner is the single most important factor that will influence the clarity and accuracy of a reading. Along with the preparation of the physical space, mental preparation is essential.

Centering

All centering techniques bring personal energies to a point of balance and rest. This helps to create enough detachment from the surroundings to create clarity of the mind, and to balance the energies of the body to encourage the easy flow of information and intuition. Here is one particularly effective centering technique.

1. Sit still for a few moments, allowing your body and breathing to settle.
2. Take your attention to your breath, and then to your spine.
3. Imagine your breath travelling up and down your spine about five to ten times.
4. Leaving the breath, direct your attention to your spine, as if it were the only part of your body.
5. After a few minutes, bring your awareness back to the present.

You can use also the "tapping-in" procedure, as described in the section on pendulum dowsing (see step 2, page 49).

Grounding

Grounding links the diviner to the resources of the planet. This connection ensures ample provision of the raw, manifesting energy necessary for a good reading. It also protects the integrity of the reader's personal energy, removing the possibility of absorbing negativity, especially when reading for someone else. Below is a time-tested technique for grounding called "growing roots."

1. Sit still for a moment or two, allowing your body and breathing to settle.
2. Direct your attention to your feet.
3. Imagine roots growing out, spreading into the earth.

4. On each out-breath, allow the roots to extend outward.
5. On each in-breath, feel the energy and stability from the earth filling the whole of your body.
6. After a minute, bring your awareness back to the present.

Grounding can be done immediately after you have centred your energy. It can also be done at any time during a reading if either party is tired or their concentration has wandered or weakened.

Dedication

Most diviners like to dedicate their work before they begin, although this is largely a matter of personal taste and conscience. In its simplest form, a dedication can be a simple request for guidance to the universe as a whole. Or, it can become as elaborate as needed. Above all, any dedication must make sense and be relevant to the diviner. If you don't adhere to any specific set of beliefs, however, then a dedication to the highest and finest energies of light may meet your needs. Whatever dedication is chosen, it must be done with awareness and faith.

Appearance

Over the years, the media have created stereotypes of clairvoyants and mediums with great panache, to the extent that the public often expects to see these people dressed in a specific costume. That said, it may well be that dressing in certain colours or styles helps create a persona that is easy to work behind.

Completion

When you have finished doing the reading, it is a good idea to have a routine that draws a clear line between reading time and everyday life.

- Centering and grounding are both essential after a reading.
- Switch off any lights of candles used.
- Fold up the board and cloth.
- Cleanse the crystals.
- Many people find it helpful to wash their hands as both a literal and symbolic gesture of separation.
- Remember to change out of "work clothes."

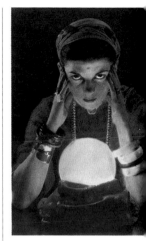

Above Adopting a dramatic appearance can set the divination session apart from everyday life, making it easier for you to work and focusing the attention of the questioner on what you are saying.

Methods of Crystal Reading

There are many ways of divining using crystals. In this section we look at some of the most popular methods: casting crystals on a divinatory board, scrying, and pendulum dowsing.

Below On the
Atlantic shores of
Europe, stone circles
were set up so that
ancient inhabitants
could accurately
predict the passage
of ritual time.

The Compass Board

The Compass board is a divinatory tool that, when crystals are cast upon it, can help clarify the questioner's present and future. When cast upon the board, the position of the fallen crystals – combined with each crystal's unique divinatory properties – are read by the diviner, who interprets them for the questioner. With this divinatory board, the directions of the compass provide the guidelines for the interpretations (see pages 52–53 for how crystals are cast, and pages 54–56 for a description of how the Compass board is used).

Evidence shows that ancient cultures found magical and ritualistic significance in the four directions of the compass. The passage of the sun through the sky was a measure of time, and the directions in which the sun and stars rose and set became an integral part of ritual and religious life. Each culture had its own descriptions of the directions, which were linked with gods and goddesses, animals, and the elements. The following descriptions are an amalgamation of Chinese, Native American, and Celtic traditions.

Northwest

This direction primarily covers social interactions and situations in which we want to help others. People who are helpful to us are shown here as well, such as those we regard as teachers or advisers – as are those who share our ideals. Social interactions may result in friction, however, so this direction can imply caution. Travel is also dealt with here.

West

Considerations of the west begin with looking after ourselves physically – taking care of our bodies. Talents that need nurturing can also make an appearance. Anything that can be considered valuable to us and which might benefit from extra care, such as children or our planet, are also placed here in the west. However, the drive to care for something can become overpowering – even destructive – if there are too many demands placed on the nurturing that we can provide. Choices can thus also be part of the west, with the added difficulty of having to choose between things we care about. The joy of living and the happiness that comes from watching those in our care flourish also belongs here.

Above The Compass Board is a tool for questioners to divine the present and future.

Southwest

The southwest covers all aspects of relationships, emphasising those with emotional ties. This is a very receptive direction, showing that we absorb emotions from others. The southwest is particularly about love – both for ourselves and for others. Love is an emotion that ebbs and flows, and requires flexibility. Even in very secure relationships, partners tend to fall in and out of love with one another continuously. The greatest challenge in a relationship is to allow the other person to be themselves. This direction is all about bringing security and trust to our relationships.

41

North

Talents come together in the north, creating the flowering of personal potential. Time and patience are needed, however, for a full realisation of this potential, and we must be able to accept and work with our own vulnerabilities and weaknesses. Without this acceptance, we have no firm ground upon which to stand.

Below The position East on the Compass board deals with family matters.

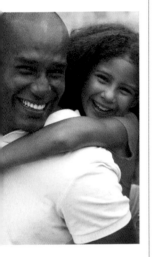

Northeast

The northeast is concerned with expanding the boundaries of knowledge. For those driven by the need to improve themselves or their situations, this direction covers education in all its forms, from day-to-day discoveries to philosophical concepts. One facet of self-improvement is taking time out to be with your own thoughts. Times of stillness and self-reflection also belong to this direction.

East

The east deals with issues surrounding the family, as well as with relationships between groups of individuals who function like a family. Questions of responsibility arise, along with the fine boundary that separates nurturing from smothering and freedom from restriction. On the negative side of the boundary, the emotional stress produced by large amounts of responsibility can cause a myriad of health problems. Changes in mental approaches to these issues can help a great deal, as can increased and more effective communication – a vital factor in healthy families.

Southeast

The southeast is associated with all aspects of wealth. Most people associate the term wealth with money, (and this direction certainly covers this form of wealth), but here we refer as well to other things that create a feeling of prosperity. For some people, this will be health, children, happiness, or friends; for others, the accumulation of possessions will suffice. This direction also relates to natural beauty, and to harmony. It can show an instinctive grasp of how life in general works, and of being in tune with the world.

South

The south is associated with recognition for the effort which we have put into our work. To achieve any level of success usually requires persistence, stubbornness, and a fair helping of luck. Faith in the workings of the world is needed to make new starts, with no certainty of the outcome. Speaking the truth is an important facet of the energies in the south. This suggestion is primarily directed toward oneself, for if a person deceives him- or herself, a price must be paid.

The Astrological Board

Based on the astrological houses, the Astrological board is another popular divinatory tool upon which crystals can be cast (see pages 50–51 for how crystals are cast, and pages 57–59 for a description of how the Astrological board is used). The astrological houses are numbered subdivisions of the astrology circle, and indicate where in an individual's life certain energies are evident. As with the Compass board, the position of the fallen crystals – combined with each crystal's divinatory properties – are read by the diviner.

Below The Astrological Board is another tool for casting crystals.

1st house

This house shows how the questioner appears to others. It can indicate as well which needs are paramount for the questioner's survival. It also shows the qualities that the questioner must learn to accept in him- or herself.

2nd house

Our values and the ways in which they shape our world are paramount in this house. These values fall into two main categories. The first category deals with the value we place on integrity, whereas the second category relates to the way we attract money and our attitude toward it.

43

3rd house

This house encompasses short journeys. It also covers the way we communicate in everyday situations. It deals as well with relationships with siblings, and also with gossip and lack of secrecy. This house also suggests adopting a more easygoing approach to life.

4th house

The roots of a problem or situation are shown here, and any hidden underlying concerns are hinted at. This house can give an indication of the emotional context of an issue, and insecurity here can lead to a great deal of fear. The home is another facet of the fourth house, so here we find residential moves and family changes. We also learn what someone expects of their home.

5th house

At first glance, this house appears to be diverse, dealing with hobbies, children, pets, creativity, romance, and gambling. However, upon closer examination, there is a uniform thread that links all of these elements: enjoyment. Here we need to lighten up, enjoy life, and take a few risks. Romantic encounters, flirting, and unconditional relationships are also included here. This house also deals with our ability to express ourselves creatively.

6th house

Everyday work situations and health are both covered by this house. The skills someone brings to their work and the type of work they enjoy are defined here. Health indications here show where the body is accumulating stress.

7th house

This house covers relationships – personal, professional, and public, and highlights relationship issues. It can also indicate the type of role someone typically plays in a public or professional context. Reactions to legal issues in a person's life are also shown here.

8th house

Situations in which deep emotions are brought to the surface are evident in this house – death, birth, or a major life change, for example. Psychic skills enabling the transference of information can also surface here. Money queries also fall within the parameters of this house.

9th house

The acquisition of knowledge is dealt with in this house. Broadcasting information through the media and learning through study or travel are all included here. Anything that extends the horizons of experience, including philosophical debate, is also present.

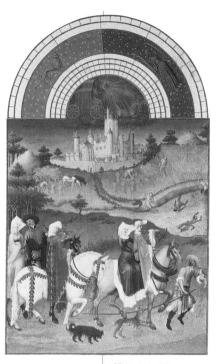

10th house

This house indicates the status of a person in the eyes of the public. It also represents the way a person wants to be seen, and thus it can actually show a self-created image. It is a vehicle for ambitions and goals, and may also show what type of long-term planning needs to be done.

11th house

Our friends and acquaintances and the activities that we enjoy in their company can be shown here. Our overall attitudes about our community are also aspects of this house, as is the willingness to serve without receiving any recognition for our efforts.

12th house

The inner realms of the individual are often evident here. This is where hidden parts of our personality can sabotage our plans. To stop this self-undoing, we need to examine our unconscious through meditation and dreams and discover what is hidden there.

Above In this fifteenth-century calendar taken from a French medieval Book of Hours, the month of August is depicted with the sun in between the first house (Aries) and the sixth house (Virgo).

45

Scrying

The crystal ball is the archetypal trademark of the fortune-teller. Scrying – the art of gazing into a crystal ball and foretelling the future – is truly a way of seeing into other worlds. The skill involves the correct interpretation of the images that appear. A ball of rock crystal or glass has typically been the favoured scrying tool, but many other items have been used as well: concave mirrors, shaped discs of black obsidian, bowls of water or ink, still pools – even thumbnails! Whatever object is used acts like a window through which the seer gazes. Scrying requires patience and persistence, but it is a useful mental exercise, even if full success is not realized.

A crystal sphere can be expensive, particularly if flawless, but it has the advantage over glass of being more conducive to stillness and a calm mind. A natural, unshaped crystal can also be used if it has a large facet that can be looked through. Obsidian spheres or large discs can also be good scrying tools. Below are some rules to follow to maximize your chances of scrying successfully.

- The scrying tool is a window upon which to rest the eyes and the mind. Set it up so that you can comfortably gaze into it without straining your body. Surrounding it with dark fabric is helpful, as this reduces the chance of distraction.
- Use subdued lighting, perhaps a candle, or even darkness. Position the scrying tool so that there are no reflections visible from where you sit.
- Close your eyes and focus on the purpose of your divination. Whatever you see or sense will in some way relate to your question, so the clearer your intention, the clearer your answer will be.
- Open your eyes and steadily gaze into the object. Do not focus on the surface, or even the interior; rather, use it as a window and look beyond it. Keep your gaze relaxed but fixed.
- With practice, a change will seem to occur after awhile. This is often described as a white mist or a swirling within the field of vision. At this point, it is important to remain

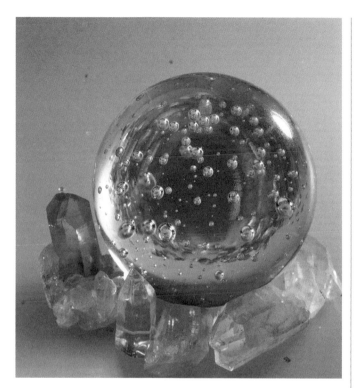

Left Whichever tool is chosen for scrying, it should help the diviner achieve an unfocused and receptive state of mind.

focused on your intention, but stay relaxed and pay close attention to everything that occurs without focusing too much on anything – like looking at the stars with your peripheral vision, or at three-dimensional computer art.

• All that is perceived is within the mind's eye rather than in the mirror or ball, and so any mental disturbance will interrupt the vision.

• When you have practiced a number of times, bring your mind back to its normal focus by covering your scrying surface with a cloth, increasing the light, and grounding yourself (see pages 38–39). Scrying creates a trance-like state, so it is important to make sure that your sense of awareness returns to its normal functioning. Make notes of your experiences.

47

Pendulum dowsing

Crystals make very useful pendulums. A pendulum works by amplifying the minuscule movements within the user to create a swing. These movements are a physical response to the subtle energy changes in the body. The types of movement the pendulum displays, particularly for yes/no responses, are individual. It can take some time to decipher pendulum responses.

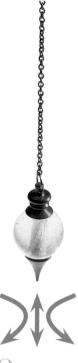

Pendulum practice

The practice exercise below is to show you that the pendulum will follow your eyes and your thoughts – if you let it. When using a pendulum to determine a yes/no response, your thoughts must be in neutral mode, and your eyes should not be focused on the pendulum; rather, they should be looking past it. If you focus your eyes directly on the pendulum and watch it closely, it will simply swing whichever way you will it to, and the divination will not be accurate.

- Find a crystal pendulum which suits you, both in terms of crystal type and weight. To find a weight of crystal with which you are comfortable, sample a selection of crystal sizes, swinging the pendulum to test how each weight feels.
- Using the arrows to the left as a guide, set the pendulum swinging over each arrow in turn, focusing on each arrow as you do so. You'll find that by watching the pendulum closely, you can will it to move in the directions of the arrows – a power you should not use when dowsing!

Finding your personal yes/no response

Having chosen a pendulum with which you would like to work, follow the steps below to determine which way your pendulum will move to indicate "yes," and which way it will move to indicate "no."

Your yes/no responses

Make a note of how the pendulum swings to indicate "yes," and how it swings to indicate "no." If both response movements look the same, don't worry. Take a break for a few hours and then try again, allowing extra time for tapping in (see step 2). You are now ready to use your pendulum as a yes/no indicator. Before you get started, however, here are a few general points to keep in mind.

• If you have too much of an emotional investment in a specific possible outcome, accurate answers are unlikely.

• The questions posed need to have "yes" or "no" as a possible answer. For example, "Is Uncle Fred's letter going to come on Monday?" If the answer is no, you would then repeat the question for each day of the week, until the answer is yes.

• If you ask a series of questions but seem to be getting nowhere, try re-examining your questions. Precise questions work best, while vague questions produce vague responses.

1. Find a place where you will have no distractions, and settle yourself into a comfortable position.
2. With either hand, tap the top of your breastbone (thymus gland) lightly with your fingertips ten to fifteen times. This action temporarily balances the energies of the body, which helps to increase the accuracy of dowsing. (This procedure is known as "tapping in.")
3. With the pendulum in one hand, set it swinging in a forward–backward movement.
4. Cover your navel with your other hand (this links you directly into the centre of the subtle energy system of the body).
5. Close your eyes.
6. Focus on the statement "Show me my 'yes' response."
7. After a short while, open your eyes and note how the pendulum is moving.
8. Repeat steps 2 through 5.
9. Focus on the statement "Show me my 'no' response."
10. After a short while, open your eyes and note the movement of the pendulum.

Facing Page A pendulum can swing in many different ways. Once you have established a clear yes/no response, you can begin to identify more subtle response movements, such as "yes, but…" or "no, but perhaps later."

49

Casting the Crystals

To make a full casting or reading, you will need at least thirteen different crystals. The stones should be no more than 25mm (an inch) in length. Once you choose your crystals, it is best if you use them for divination only; this way, you will ensure that your readings maintain their sacredness and purity. Each time the stones are used, it is important to cleanse them.

Casting can involve letting the crystals fall at random over the board, or it can mean placing them specifically and deliberately onto areas of the board. If the stones are thrown and some fall off of the board, this has implications for the interpretation. Here are some commonly used methods of casting crystals on a board.

Shake and throw

Select a total of thirteen crystals from the stones that are available to you. You can include your personal stone in this number (see pages 30–35), or select thirteen stones in addition to your personal stone. If the crystals are small enough, collect them in your hands and gently shake them. While you are doing this, focus your thoughts on the question at hand. When the time feels right, release the crystals onto the board. Leave all of the stones where they land.

Casting can involve letting the crystals fall at random over the board, or it can mean placing them specifically and deliberately onto areas of the board. If the stones are thrown and some fall off of the board, this has implications for the interpretation. Here are some commonly used methods of casting crystals on a board.

Casting one by one

Have your crystals close at hand, but keep them out of your direct sight, in a bag or box. Focus on the question at hand. Pick one crystal and cast it onto the board. Repeat this process until you have a total of twelve or thirteen crystals on the board. Cast your personal stone last. With this method, the subconscious mind adjusts slightly as each selection is made. This adjustment lends the reading a greater depth and accuracy, particularly if the issue is complex.

Individual placement
Take a moment to focus on the empty board with your question in mind. Taking your focus to the first area where you want to place a stone – perhaps the area most relevant to the issue – pick a stone at random and place it within that area. Continue using the same procedure until every desired area has had a stone placed upon it. If your personal crystal is among your selections, place it in the centre to complete the spread, or place it intuitively in one of the sections, for extra focus.

Targeted reading
Referring to the crystal information pages contained herein (see pages 60–213), choose the thirteen stones that seem to best reflect the subject matter that is relevant to your question. These stones can be cast randomly onto the board, or you can use the individual placement method.

Below Make sure your board is placed upon a surface that is large enough to catch any stones that may fall off the board when cast randomly.

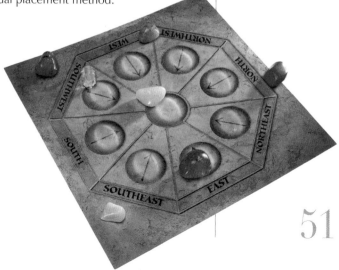

51

Interpreting the Crystals

Interpretation in any type of reading will make sense only if the question posed is kept in mind during the entire process, so that the information given relates to the relevant issue. For example, if the reading is about work, but it is interpreted in terms of romance, it will not be helpful, and will likely be misleading.

The person doing the reading must sift through several possible interpretations of the reading, and then ascertain which interpretation is the relevant (i.e. correct) one for the questioner. The decision as to which interpretation is relevant is an intuitive one, and may be made by the diviner alone or in conjunction with the questioner. It is important to recognise that there is seldom a right or wrong interpretation, just different degrees of possibility.

Both the Compass and Astrological boards have their own key words, as do each of the crystals. When you begin to interpret a reading, start by putting the relevant sets of key words together. Both boards will tell you where in the life of the questioner the relevant energy or issue is likely to appear, while each of the crystals will explain which energy or issue is being highlighted. Don't be disheartened if at first you find it hard to blend the key words together. The more readings you do, the easier reading becomes, and the more meanings you will be able to incorporate. When using either board, it is a good idea to keep a written record of the question posed. This will help keep you focused, and will insure that your questions are concise.

Crystal groupings

To refine your reading of the crystals, you should bear in mind certain supplementary insights offered by the positions of the crystals that have been randomly cast on the board. The following rules apply to crystals cast on both the Compass and Astrological boards.

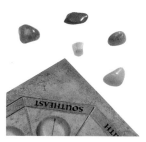

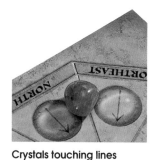

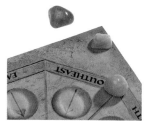

Crystals falling some distance off the board: The energies suggested by these crystals are not at issue at this particular time, but may be more appropriate in about three months' time.

Crystals touching lines between directions or houses: These crystals will have influence in both areas they touch, so both will need to be considered.

Crystals falling just off the board: The energies of these crystals are on the periphery of the question, and are likely to be part of the picture in two weeks' time.

Crystals over the edge of the board circle, partly in: These are influences incoming or outgoing during the next week; intuition may indicate which.

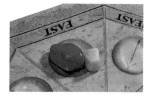

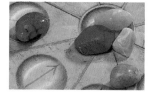

Crystals touching each other in the same section: These crystals are inextricably linked together, and need to be interpreted as such.

Crystals falling at the centre and/or touching the personal stone, if used: These crystals are tied in very closely with the questioner, and will represent very personal characteristics.

Groups of crystals: Where a bunch of crystals land in a group, the area that they occupy is emphasised.

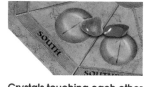

Crystals touching each other in different sections: Both sections are seen as linked together through each of the crystal energies.

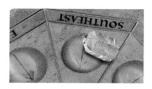

Crystals that are long and thin: These suggest linkage between the sections of the board they point toward.

53

Interpreting the Compass Board

For those who are beginners at casting, the crystals on the board, once cast, can seem confusing, and their interpretation may seem like an overwhelming task. It is thus advisable to read the crystals in the sequence that appears below, starting from the south and ending with southeast. As you become more familiar with the board, and with the various ways in which the directions interact with the crystals, you will probably develop your own reading sequence.

See page 53 for the meaning of crystals that fall in the following ways:
- outside the boundaries of the board or partly in
- on lines between directions or houses
- touching each other in the same or different sections
- at the centre of the board
- touching your personal stone
- pointing in a certain direction
- in groups

See also pages 60–213 for interpretations of specific crystals cast upon the board.

South
Crystals that land here show how to gain recognition. In questions concerning romance, look for crystals indicating persistence: these can help to get a relationship moving. Blue crystals here show a need to let things flow. Red crystals suggest the need to begin again.
Key words: Recognition, luck, beginnings, honesty

Southwest

Crystals that land here describe facets of any sort of relationship. Pink crystals address the questioner's input into the situation, whereas green crystals hint at the quality of the relationship.

Key words: Relationships, receptivity, flexibility, compassion, possessiveness

West

Crystals landing here highlight our capacity to fulfil our daily needs. This can extend to people or relationships that are in need of nurturing. Black, red, or clear crystals here may suggest that priorities need to be re-examined. Yellow or gold crystals hint at the need to develop personal skills.

Key words: Caring, physical needs, children, talents, pleasure

Northwest

The northwest covers friends and community. Violet and pink crystals will point to areas where others may be helped; blue crystals suggest that the questioner seek expert advice. Arguments between friends can also show up here, especially when black or red crystals are present. Any crystal can indicate travel.

Key words: Service, adviser, travel, friends, disagreements

North

The north deals with the integration of various threads of an issue to reach a successful conclusion. Crystals falling here will indicate the fruits of hard work. Certain crystals can hint at personal tendencies that may inhibit success unless watched. Yellow and blue crystals indicate the need to share knowledge.

Key words: Career, wisdom, going with the flow, security, perceived weakness

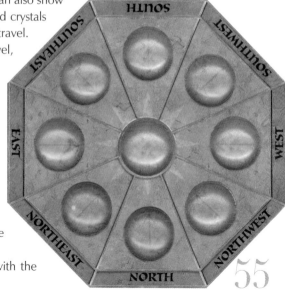

55

Northeast

Crystals landing here pinpoint what is needed to improve a situation; the specific crystals will indicate what needs to be done. For example, yellow or clear stones show that more information is needed. Crystals that land here can also help to answer questions regarding love or illness.

Key words: Education, self-development, stillness, respite

East

All familial issues are anchored here. Green and red crystals indicate the need to respect other people's space; blue and yellow stones show a need to communicate. Black, red, and clear stones hint at issues that need attention. Violet and pink crystals suggest health concerns.

Key words: Family, relationships, responsibility, health, personal boundaries

Southeast

If the question concerns money, this is the area to watch. Yellow and green crystals represent an added bonus, even if the overall reading appears negative. That which is needed to feel wealthy, be it money, health, or love, is likely to be shown here.

Key words: Wealth, prosperity, harmony

Interpreting the Astrological Board

As with the Compass board, beginner casters are best off reading the crystals in the sequence that appears below, starting from the 1st house and ending with the 12th house. This systematic approach will help prevent confusion.

See page 53 for the meaning of crystals that fall in the following ways:
- outside the boundaries of the board or partly in
- on lines between directions or houses
- touching each other in the same or different sections
- at the centre of the board
- touching your personal stone
- pointing in a certain direction
- in groups

See also pages 60–213 for interpretations of specific crystals cast upon the board.

1st house

Crystals that land here will indicate first impressions of a situation. Any considerations that the questioner should examine will be highlighted here.

Key words: Appearances, individuality

2nd house

Issues surrounding money need to be closely examined. Black, clear, or red crystals can point to changes needed. Blue or green crystals here focus on truth and hint that motives and honesty are in question.

Key words: Money, possessions, values

3rd house

Crystals landing here relate to communication. Clear, yellow, or gold crystals indicate a need for precision. Black, brown, and red crystals show that confusion is creating difficulties. Family considerations are present if green crystals appear. Any crystal may signal travel.

Key words: Communication, family, gossip, travel

4th house

The crystals that land here will clarify the situation at hand. Problems in the questioner's life can show up here. Look for situations that are fuelling insecurity. Blue crystals suggest the need for independence. Orange, gold, or red crystals show that action is needed.

Key words: Home, roots, family, stability, protection

5th house

Any crystal here suggests that more leisure time is needed. Green or blue crystals hint that more time should be spent outdoors. Pink, green, and red crystals indicate romance. Black crystals suggest undiscovered skills.

Key words: Creativity, romance, leisure

6th house

This house deals with work and health matters. Clear or white crystals suggest that a readjustment of the situation at hand is needed to remedy matters. Violet crystals emphasise the healing facets of a question.

Key words: Work, healing, service, health issues, crisis points

7th house

Crystals here suggest the existence of issues surrounding long-term relationships. Green crystals indicate a need to examine the balance of relationships. Black, clear, or red crystals hint at changing dynamics.

Key words: Relationships, partnerships

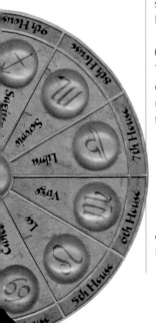

8th house

This house can emphasise psychic input, especially if violet, dark blue, or black stones land here. The appearance of more than one crystal indicates that an event has been delayed. If the question involves money, green or gold crystals suggest the need for a decision.
Key words: Finance, endings, beginnings, subtle forces, deep emotions

9th house

Crystal energies here are a means to extend existing knowledge into new areas. The appearance of more than one stone shows that the questioner's outlook is too narrow. Any crystal here can indicate travel. Blue and yellow crystals call attention to learning.
Key words: Education, travel, broadcasting, philosophy, expansion

10th house

This house deals with the culmination of something – a career, a relationship, or a project. Crystals landing here show the factors affecting that outcome. They can also indicate how the questioner wants to be seen by others. Goals can also be shown here.
Key words: Career, ambition, status, planning

11th house

The influence of friends is shown here. Blue crystals indicate the need to reassess what is really going on and to ascertain who is influencing the questioner. Pink crystals show the need to be more compassionate with acquaintances.
Key words: Friends, social life, group issues, ideals

12th house

Interpretation of crystals here may be difficult. Red crystals suggest the need for action. All other crystals indicate areas that should be explored in the questioner's life. Most insights illuminated here involve areas of self-sabotage as a result of personal beliefs.
Key words: Introspection, silence, self-sabotage

OUTHWEST

9th House

8th House

The Crystal Directory

In the pages that follow, crystals are the tools of divination. The meanings given to each of the forty-five featured crystals are derived from their unique physical characteristics, historical uses, mythical attributes, and spiritual and healing properties, all of which are described for each crystal. Sample readings for the placement of each crystal on both the Compass and Astrological boards are also provided, to help you determine which energies are at play. The crystals in the following section are ordered by colour, clear through to black.

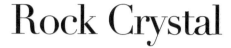

Rock Crystal

Rock crystal is the common name for transparent, clear quartz. This stone has been used for thousands of years for both healing and prophecy.

Clear quartz is the pure form of the mineral silicon dioxide. It is free of any impurity in the crystal lattice that might create colour, and forms long, hexagonal crystals that meet at a single point. It originates in volcanic rock, where silica-rich solutions cool and crystallise within cracks and cavities. A hard-wearing stone, quartz finds its way via eroded material into sedimentary layers, rivers, and seabeds. The great majority of beach pebbles are quartz varieties, and sand itself is mostly silicate minerals.

Myth and history

In ancient Greece, there were some who believed that clear quartz was ice that had frozen so completely that it would never melt again, *crystallos* being the Greek word for ice. Other ancient peoples associated quartz with the sky worlds, and saw it as fragments from the heavenly realms.

Historically, quartz was universally used as a tool for divination, scrying, and healing – particularly for divining the causes of disease and for the removal of imbalances caused by the spirits. Clear quartz was one of the favourite materials for fashioning mirrors and spheres for scrying. It was also ground into lenses and cut to make goblets and bowls for ritual purposes. Among the most famous of quartz carvings are the crystal skulls attributed to the ancient cultures of South and Central America.

Rock crystal

Colour: transparent, clear
Hardness: 7
Composition: SiO_2
Qualities: clear, orderly, calm
Main chakra: all

Suggested Crystal Readings

Rock crystal in centre/First House
Be yourself. Let others see how you really feel.

Rock crystal in southeast/Second House
Doubts need to be resolved if you are going to make progress.

Rock crystal in east/Third House
Explain things carefully to others, repeating yourself until you are sure they understand.

Rock crystal in north/Fourth House
Issues surrounding the home and family cannot be ignored any longer.

Rock crystal in west/Fifth House
It is not a good time to take risks or to gamble. Stick with what you are sure of.

Rock crystal in Sixth House
This is an ideal time to resolve difficulties in the workplace.

Rock crystal in southwest/Seventh House
Pretence should have no place in your relationships or partnerships.

Rock crystal in Eighth House
Financial dealings need to be honest and transparent.

Rock crystal in northeast/Ninth House
Your perception of current circumstances is particularly clear at the moment – be guided by it.

Rock crystal in south/Tenth House
Your plans need to be clear and open to scrutiny by others.

Rock crystal in northwest/Eleventh House
A frank exchange of ideas may help to clarify problems or disagreements.

Rock crystal in Twelfth House
You need to be sure that you are not working to a hidden agenda that is clouding the issue.

Crystals are placed on all the chakras.

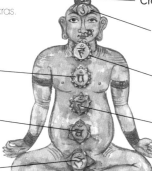

Crown chakra top of the head

Brow chakra centre of forehead

Heart chakra centre of breastbone in centre of chest

Throat chakra neck

Sacral chakra midway between navel and pubic bone

Solar Plexus chakra midway between navel and base of ribs

Base (root) chakra base of spine (perineum)

Right Many instances of healing and otherworldly communications have been attributed to ancient crystal skulls.

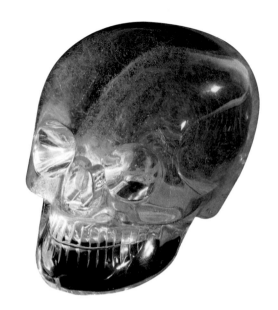

In the development of modern technology, quartz crystal has been vital. For example, tons of Brazilian quartz was mined during World War II for radio sets. Quartz is also widely used as a component in precision equipment, although laboratory-made crystals are now the main source for the industry.

Personality

Rock crystal indicates a bright, organised, orderly individual with a calm, clear mind and a positive emotional outlook..

Energy

Clear, transparent, coherent.

Spiritual and healing properties

Rock crystal has an organising and harmonising effect on all parts of the body with which it comes into contact. It can be especially calming, and will quickly restore a more balanced energy. It also helps to dissipate all areas of imbalance and negativity, and establishes calmness and clarity in the mind, making it a useful stone for meditation and healing techniques.

Rock crystal tends to amplify the qualities of stones nearby. It will also amplify positive frequencies of energy, making coherent, life-enhancing energies more effective, while reducing or neutralising chaotic or unharmonious ones.

Divinatory interpretation

Rock crystal acts as a focus for solidity and organisation in a reading, and brings clarity and understanding. It helps keep necessary information out in the open, and ensures that nothing is withheld or disguised. All activities will tend to be productive and helpful in the areas where rock crystal falls. Only when the questioner is planning some sort of subterfuge or secret dealings will this stone indicate a failure of plans; this is because everything will become transparent and obvious to all involved.

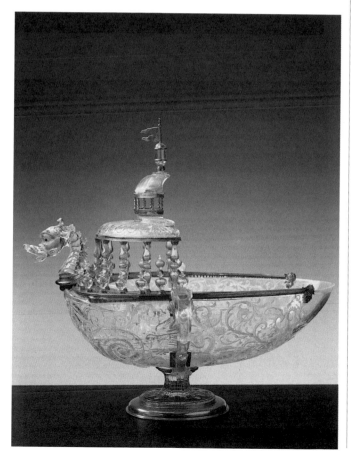

Left Before the advent of electric light, rock crystal was often used to reflect candlelight in candelabra and table fountains. This rock crystal and gold table fountain was made specially for the Medici family.

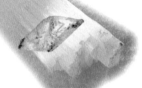

Selenite

Selenite is named for the ancient Greek goddess of the moon, Selene, because of its gentle white lustre.

Selenite is the transparent, gem-quality variety of the common mineral gypsum. It forms long, blade-like crystals made up of parallel sheets of rock. Gypsum is extremely soft and can be easily scratched. It is formed from the evaporation of saltwater lakes and ancient seas.

Myth and history

Selenite
Colour: transparent, white, grey
Hardness: 2
Composition: $CaSO_4 2H_2O$
(gypsum variety)
Qualities: energy-shifting, expansive
Main chakra: crown, sacral

The extreme delicacy of selenite severely limits its use – the stone has a high water content, and exposure to heat or a change of humidity can bend the crystals. If left in water for too long, selenite can easily separate into thin leaves.

The Greek sculptor Lysippus is said to have been the first to use gypsum as a casting material. Today, its use for casting is widespread, and is commonly known as plaster of Paris. Plaster of Paris is gypsum heated to about 4,000°C (7,230°F), to drive out the water (once water is reintroduced, the material recrystallises). When heated above this temperature, gypsum is suitable for making paint bulkers and cement. The fine, granular, massive form of gypsum is known as alabaster, and is an important sculpting material.

Spiritual and healing properties

Selenite is one of the best stones with which to bring about a rapid shift of energy. It can quickly disperse accumulations of negativity in the aura, and will remove blockages and stagnant energy from the body. Selenite also brings flexibility, spiritual insight, and creativity. It can be relaxing and eases bodily tension.

Suggested Crystal Readings

Selenite in centre/First House
Be flexible and philosophical, as there is little you can do about the situation.

Selenite in southeast/Second House
Trying to keep to a routine is likely to be pointless at the moment.

Selenite in east/Third House
Other people's reactions show you how delicate circumstances are at present.

Selenite in north/Fourth House
You may be feeling sorry for yourself, but this will pass.

Selenite in west/Fifth House
Soft music and gentle relaxation in beautiful surroundings are needed now.

Selenite in Sixth House
Your health may not be at its most robust, so take it easy for a while.

Selenite in southwest/Seventh House
Be sympathetic to those close to you – listen but do not react.

Selenite in Eighth House
Others' emotions are deeply connected here, so be prepared for sudden changes.

Selenite in northeast/Ninth House
Life is likely to feel like a rollercoaster ride, so just let go and flow with it.

Selenite in south/Tenth House
The current situation is too unstable to make plans for the future.

Selenite in northwest/Eleventh House
For the next few weeks, group situations could be very finely balanced, so respond with care.

Selenite in Twelfth House
Keep your feet on the ground and try not to get carried away with whims and illusions.

Personality
Watch out for the selenite personality. They may appear attractive and friendly, but in reality they can be unreliable and unstable.

Energy
Fluctuating, vulnerable.

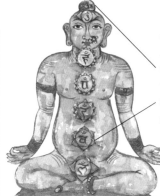

Crystals are placed on the crown and sacral chakras.
Crown chakra top of the head
Sacral chakra midway between navel and pubic bone

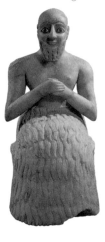

Divinatory interpretation

When it appears in a reading, selenite suggests that the situation is extremely delicate. On the surface, things may appear to be fine, with nothing apparently amiss. In reality, however, the situation is inherently unstable. This doesn't necessarily mean that things are going to get worse, but it does mean that some sort of change lies ahead. As selenite is associated with the moon, and the cycle of the moon is around twenty-eight days, it may be that change will occur within a month of the day of the reading. Precisely what that change will be may be indicated by the fall of other stones, or by the area occupied by selenite in the cast.

Selenite will indicate problems in a reading only if the questioner is unwilling to face change in the area of his or her life to which it relates. In a situation that is difficult or blocked, selenite provides instant relief by allowing the energies involved to move once more. Once circumstances begin to change, there will be a rapid alteration in all lives involved.

Selenite in a personal placement suggests that the questioner move very carefully, as he or she is extremely vulnerable. Negative emotions such as anger and fear should be allowed to dissolve before they precipitate unexpected and unwelcome responses. In partnerships, selenite can indicate the need to maintain sympathetic and open conditions. Any change now may result in one stress too many and lead to a parting of ways.

68

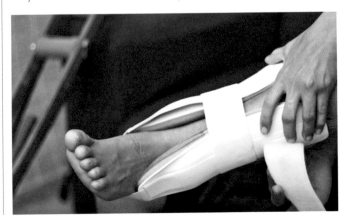

Labradorite

Labradorite is a chameleon like
stone, ranging from the dullest of
greys to peacock iridescence as
it catches the light.

L abradorite is a special variety of feldspar. Large areas of the stone are exceptionally iridescent. The colour is caused by light refracting from microscopic crystals of various dark minerals, usually ilmenite, hematite, and magnetite, and from fine intergrowths of labradorite crystals. It is common in massive form; crystals are rare and small. Labradorite is found in both igneous and metamorphic conditions.

Myth and history

In the late eighteenth century, a missionary exploring the shores of Labrador found boulders of this strange mineral. Soon after this initial identification, labradorite was found in Finland and the Ukraine, although Labrador remained the primary source for gem-quality stone. The beauty of the stone ensured that it quickly became favoured for carving ornaments and jewellery.

Spiritual and healing properties

Labradorite allows complete polarity shifts to occur. Just as different colours appear on the surface of the stone, so the stone helps many different levels of energy and awareness to be accessed by the individual. Because of this quality, it can be an ideal stone to help discover new solutions and reveal new opportunities in life.

Labradorite

Colour: grey with blue, green, and orange iridescence
Hardness: 6
Composition: $(Na,Ca)Al_{1-2}Si_{3-2}2O_8$ (plagioclase feldspar)
Qualities: camouflage, energy-shifting
Main chakra: all

69

Suggested Crystal Readings

Labradorite in centre/First House
You need to stand firm and not be swayed by the dominant view.

Labradorite in southeast/Second House
Look at ways of eliminating waste and unnecessary pressures from your life.

Labradorite in east/Third House
Choices should be intuitive rather than based on intellectual thought.

Labradorite in north/Fourth House
Consider rearranging things at home to create a sense of more space and light.

Labradorite in west/Fifth House
Try to do more outdoors, in a natural environment.

Labradorite in Sixth House
Look after your health, especially if demanding people surround you.

Labradorite in southwest/Seventh House
Make the most of your relationships and partnerships.

Labradorite in Eighth House
It is time to transform or release old situations.

Labradorite in northeast/Ninth House
Unexpected opportunities may change your view of the situation.

Labradorite in south/Tenth House
Old plans and ideas may once again be relevant, and may need to be relaunched.

Labradorite in northwest/Eleventh House
Don't take your friends for granted. Find a way to show your appreciation for them.

Labradorite in Twelfth House
Quiet times will help you regain your energy and enthusiasm.

Crystals are placed on all of the chakras.

Heart chakra centre of breastbone in centre of chest

Sacral chakra midway between navel and pubic bone

Crown chakra top of the head

Brow chakra centre of forehead

Throat chakra neck

Solar Plexus chakra midway between navel and base of ribs

Base (root) chakra base of spine (perineum)

The ability of labradorite to instigate rapid frequency shifts enables the body chakras to move easily between dimensional states. This can remove blockages rapidly, and can help to establish new patterns of behaviour that are more appropriate to the individual.

Labradorite is a very useful stone for energy protection, as the ever-changing colours prevent negativity from attaching to any one place. It also prevents energy drainage and reduces co-dependency.

Personality

This crystal represents a seemingly dull, boring person who, as you suddenly discover, has always had – unbeknownst to you – a much more exciting life than you have!

Energy

Transformative, surprising, unexpected.

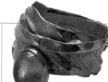

Divinatory interpretation

Labradorite indicates surprise, transformation, and transmutation. It brings a sudden change of circumstances that enables a stagnant situation to revive and move on in a positive way. New opportunities will arise, a variety of choices will present themselves, and life will suddenly become full of excitement and opportunity.

The lesson of this stone is never to make assumptions. In relationships, labradorite can indicate the need to look carefully at what you have; taking the situation for granted creates boredom and a stifling routine. Do something unnecessary, unexpected, and generous. Show your appreciation for your partner.

If labradorite is found in a position of health, it may show the need to monitor personal energies. Do you always feel drained in the presence of some people, and do those people feel better for being with you? If you work with many people all day long, or are in a stressful occupation where emotions can be strongly broadcast, labradorite can indicate that your energy is not being replenished sufficiently, and that you are accumulating stress.

Above Wearing labradorite can provide a boost of energy for those who tire easily in the company of others.

Left Like the metamorphosis of a caterpillar into a butterfly, labradorite can transform stagnant, dull energies into fresh, vibrant ones, and can signal the advent of brand new beginnings.

71

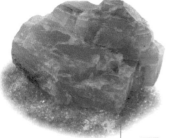

Moonstone

Moonstone has a soft blue-white sheen that is reminiscent of the gentle light cast by the moon.

Moonstone is the generic name given to a number of related minerals with similar appearances. All moonstones belong to the oligoclase family of feldspars, and are the purest members of this mineral family originating from hot solutions.

Feldspar is one of the most common minerals on the planet. Often displaying interesting plays of light within the crystal structure, it is composed of parallel layers of mineral that reflect the light entering the crystal. Moonstone is unique in its soft iridescence.

Myth and history

Fine crystals of nearly transparent moonstone are commonly found throughout the Mont Blanc mountain range. In fact, another name for moonstone is adularia; this name is derived from Mount Adula, near St. Gotthard, in Switzerland, where moonstone is often found. However, it is in India that moonstone has had the longest history. Indian women in particular have long held the stone in high esteem. Not only is it thought to emphasise female virtues, but it is also believed to help alleviate assorted digestive problems, as well as reproductive ailments afflicting women in particular.

Moonstone
Colour: pearly white, yellow, blue
Hardness: 6-6.5
Composition: $KAlSi_3O_8$
(potassium aluminum silicate)
Qualities: emotionally balancing, intuitive, calming
Main chakra: solar plexus, sacral

Spiritual and healing properties

Moonstone is one of the best stones for bringing emotional calm and stability, as it has the ability to quickly release tensions created by emotional stress. This stress often affects the

Suggested Crystal Readings

Moonstone in centre/First House
You need to be more approachable and receptive.

Moonstone in southeast/Second House
Learn to trust your gut feelings and stick by them.

Moonstone in east/Third House
You are very intuitive, but you should keep your observations to yourself.

Moonstone in north/Fourth House
There are emotional undercurrents in your family. Tread carefully.

Moonstone in west/Fifth House
Time spent by the sea or near a river will help settle your emotions.

Moonstone in Sixth House
Health problems are likely affecting your digestion.

Moonstone in southwest/Seventh House
Relationships are being clouded by emotions at this time.

Moonstone in Eighth House
Beginnings and endings are a natural part of life. Learn to accept this reality.

Moonstone in northeast/Ninth House
Allow time to absorb new information before acting on it or passing it on to others.

Moonstone in south/Tenth House
Do not rush into anything at this time. Wait at least three days before taking action.

Moonstone in northwest/Eleventh House
Listen to what your friends and acquaintances say before acting.

Moonstone in Twelfth House
You may find yourself easily swayed by other people's strong opinions or feelings.

Crystals are placed on the solar plexus and sacral chakras.

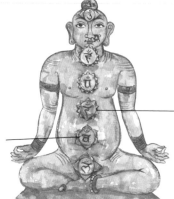

Solar plexus chakra midway between navel and base of ribs

Sacral chakra midway between navel and pubic bone

73

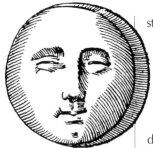

stomach and digestive system, disrupting normal processes of absorbing nutrition from food. Stomachaches and headaches can also be relieved if their source is emotional.

Just as the moon itself has a relationship with water, moods, cycles, and intuition, so does moonstone encourage a fluidity and flexibility in all body systems. Fluid balance can be restored, as can body cycles that have been disrupted through shock and stress. All problems involving the flow of energy, particularly in the female reproductive system, can be eased. Intuition, creativity, and empathy can also increase with moonstone.

Divinatory interpretation

Moonstone has a very feminine energy, and thus, in a reading, it can represent an important female in the questioner's life. It can also stand for the feminine qualities of empathy, listening, and sensitivity.

This stone shows that emotional balance is needed in a situation. Stress may be building up, creating a rigidity in relationships that needs to be loosened. When moonstone falls in an area relating to health, it signals that emotional stress may be creating stomachaches, digestive problems, or headaches.

Moonstone also indicates a need for intuitive skills. Now is not the time for strident action – observe, feel, and sense what

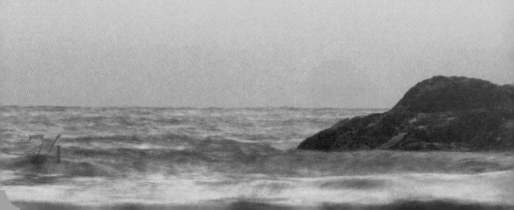

is going on within you and around you before you do anything. There are delicate creative energies coming together at this time, and so it is best to proceed with patience and care.

Because the moon controls so many of the life cycles on our planet, moonstone in a reading may indicate that the questioner should be aware that there is a natural cycle of growth to all things. There is no point in trying to rush things – everything happens in its own time.

Personality

Moonstone suggests a personality with strong feminine qualities, though not necessarily a woman.

Energy

Emotionally balanced, intuitive, cyclical.

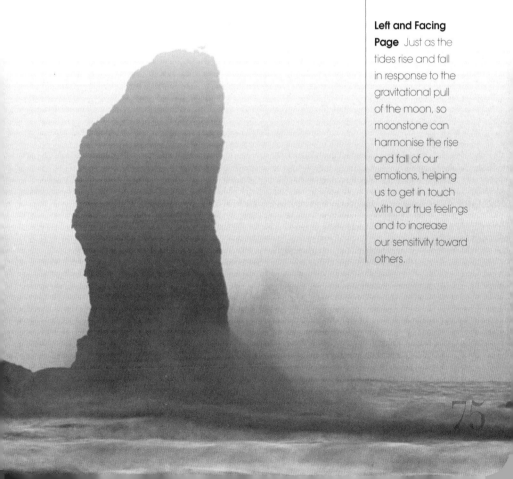

Left and Facing Page Just as the tides rise and fall in response to the gravitational pull of the moon, so moonstone can harmonise the rise and fall of our emotions, helping us to get in touch with our true feelings and to increase our sensitivity toward others.

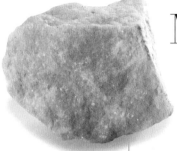

Milky Quartz

Milky quartz is a cloudy type of rock crystal that contains a myriad of tiny gas or water bubbles.

Many types of rock crystal contain veins and patterns of small bubbles within their clear, transparent interiors, usually caused by water or gas. The base of quartz crystals is often cloudy, with small bubbles; this cloudy section is called milky quartz. Milky quartz can sometimes turn clear when gentle warmth is applied.

Myth and history

Less precious than the transparent variety, milky quartz has not had as exalted a history, but it has been used for making beads for jewellery for some time. It also has a long history of use for demarcating special or sacred spaces. Many megalithic sites in Western Europe have stones with a high milky quartz content. At Newgrange, a megalithic burial site in Ireland built around 3200 BC, the large central ceremonial chamber was given an outer covering of white quartz walls.

Spiritual and healing properties

Milky quartz has all the same energies as clear quartz, except that it has a more gentle, feminine effect. Just as it gently diffuses light, so it softly radiates a cool, quiet energy into the aura.

Milky quartz is soothing to both the mind and the emotions. It blends all energies around it together, and has a gentle, purifying effect. It is like rose quartz in many ways, but without the focus on emotional states.

Milky quartz

Colour: opaque white, translucent
Hardness: 7
Composition: SiO_2
Qualities: gentle diffusion, dispersal
Main chakra: sacral, crown

Suggested Crystal Readings

Milky quartz in centre/First House
Your question is not clear – try again with a more focused question.

Milky quartz in southeast/Second House
Keep a tight reign on your finances over the next few days.

Milky quartz in east/Third House
You need to be precise when asking others to follow your instructions.

Milky quartz in north/Fourth House
Stay at home, sit quietly, and relax.

Milky quartz in west/Fifth House
Now is not the time to focus on any one project.

Milky quartz in Sixth House
This is not a good time for decisions – wait until the picture is clearer.

Milky quartz in southwest/Seventh House
Relationships may seem insubstantial and unstable at present.

Milky quartz in Eighth House
The timing of events is likely to be erratic or vague, so don't rely too heavily on a rigid schedule.

Milky quartz in northeast/Ninth House
Share your ideas and skills as much as possible.

Milky quartz in south/Tenth House
Your current plans may become irrelevant as the situation develops.

Milky quartz in northwest/Eleventh House
People around you may be confused or annoyed by your lack of clarity.

Milky quartz in Twelfth House
You should not trust your feelings about people or events at the moment.

Personality
Milky quartz characterises a rather vague, unfocused individual; he or she is well-meaning, but is not particularly effective in everyday life.

Energy
Vague, confused.

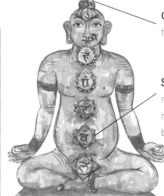

Crown chakra
top of the head

Sacral chakra
midway between navel and pubic bone

77

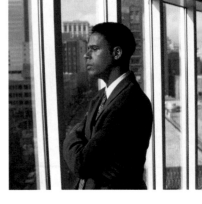

Divinatory interpretation

Milky quartz in a reading indicates that there is some lack of definition or clarity in the situation. This may be causing some frustration, but now is simply not the time to act. Patience is required for the gentle, dissipating effects of milky quartz to bring clarity to the situation.

Keep in mind that a lack of focus may be advantageous in some circumstances – it offers a rest from continuous attention to detail. At any rate, for better or worse, nothing much can be achieved, whether the fogginess is in the mind of the questioner or the surrounding events. It is best to just relax and wait for clarity.

If milky quartz falls in the section that relates to the main thrust of the question, this may suggest that the question itself is lacking in clarity. If this is felt to be the case, rethink your wording or approach and ask the question again.

When milky quartz falls amongst stones of conflict, this suggests that the situation will lose its internal energy naturally, and the negativity will disperse on its own. If found near strong stones, milky quartz will diffuse some of their energy, but it will also help to integrate any conflicting patterns in the way the stones have fallen.

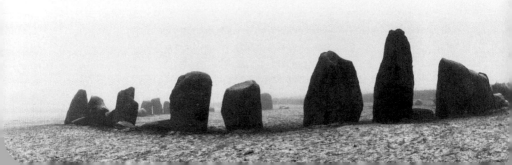

Pearl/Abalone

Both pearl and abalone shell are organic gemstones derived from shellfish.

Pearl and abalone shell are variable compounds, but are both basically comprised of the same mineral: calcium carbonate. (The gemstones aragonite and calcite are also made of this compound in inorganic form.)

Pearls form inside the shells of certain molluscs in both the sea and in fresh water as a response to the irritation of grains of sand or parasites. Their iridescence is caused by light dispersing from the microcrystals of calcium carbonate. Abalone is a widespread, edible shellfish that has an inner shell with many shiny, iridescent colours, mainly blues and greens.

Myth and history

The name "pearl" is thought to derive from the Latin word pernula, the diminuitive of the word perna, meaning "sea shell" or "mussel."

Pearl is a very soft gemstone with little resistance to impact, chemicals, or drying conditions, but it has always been regarded as one of the most precious of jewels for its rarity and beauty. Traditionally, perfectly clear, unblemished, round pearls were the primary gemstone of the moon in India. When set in silver, they were thought to remove problems caused by an inauspicious placement of the moon in one's natal chart. In both India and China, the pearl is the epitome and symbol of purity, excellence, longevity, immortality, enlightenment, and wisdom.

Abalone shell is much more robust than pearl, and has been used in many cultures as a decoration for inlays into carvings

Pearl
Colour: white, pink, brown, black
Hardness: 2.5–3.5
Composition: $CaCO_3$ + conchiolin + H_2O
Qualities: tolerant, flexibile
Main chakra: sacral

Abalone
Colour: iridescent blues, greens, silver, red
Hardness: 3.5–4
Composition: variable $CaCO_3$
Qualities: flexible, immune
Main chakra: heart, sacral

Suggested Crystal Readings

Pearl/abalone in centre/First House
You need to place family concerns first on your priority list.

Pearl/abalone in southeast/Second House
Don't rely on resources that you don't actually possess or own.

Pearl/abalone in east/Third House
Try to be sensitive and delicate in your communications.

Pearl/abalone in north/Fourth House
Look to the women in your family for guidance and support.

Pearl/abalone in west/Fifth House
Appreciate the beauty of the situation and try to adjust.

Pearl/abalone in Sixth House
Be flexible to events at work and tune in to underlying emotions.

Pearl/abalone in southwest/Seventh House
Try to be sensitive and patient with the moods of those around you.

Pearl/abalone in Eighth House
Family or relationship issues from the past may resurface.

Pearl/abalone in northeast/Ninth House
Don't commit yourself to any specific viewpoint or stance – keep an open mind.

Pearl/abalone in south/Tenth House
No single path to the future can be guaranteed given the present fluctuation in events.

Pearl/abalone in northwest/Eleventh House
Friends may need consoling or nurturing, and may look to you.

Pearl/abalone in Twelfth House
Spend some time by the sea or watching the cycle of the moon in order to reconnect to nature's energies.

Crystals are placed on the heart and sacral chakras.

Heart chakra centre of breastbone in centre of chest

Sacral chakra midway between navel and pubic bone

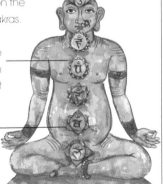

Personality
Pearl and abalone personalities may be outwardly beautiful and inwardly confused. A great deal of emotional energy exists. However, if there is no balancing factor, this may lead to instability.

Energy
Sensitive, family-oriented, confused.

and for jewellery. A disc of abalone shell is worn on the forehead of Apache girls as they greet the sun on the morning of their initiation into womanhood.

Mother-of-pearl is made of essentially the same material as abalone shell and pearl. It is the thick layer on the inner surface of shells from which pearls are grown – hence its common name. It is also known as "nacre."

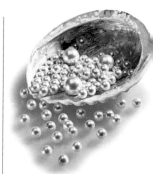

Spiritual and healing properties

Pearl is thought to be the finest stabiliser of the emotions. It increases tolerance and flexibility, and brings relaxation where there has been tension and frustration. Digestive functions are eased, and there is an increase in self-assuredness. All functions of a watery nature or involving a flow of some sort within the body are regulated by pearl.

Abalone strengthens the structure of the body and the functions of the heart chakra. Increased emotional expression and a strengthening of the immune system can also be expected. As well, abalone encourages individuality and expansion.

Above Pearls with a perfect lustre and shape are rare, making the best specimens very costly.

Divinatory interpretation

Both pearl and abalone shell have the same divinatory meanings: they are intimately connected to the sea, and to the tides of the emotions. An easy flow of feelings, sensitivity to others, and awareness of personal needs are all indicated in a positive, balanced reading. Very often, these gems will represent the family, particularly the mother. Their highly changeable colouration suggests that, like our human emotions, matters are in a state of continual flux. Life is all about change, and these gems remind us that nothing stays the same for long – especially where the emotions are concerned. Like the play of colours in pearl and abalone, change is the beauty of existence.

In places where these gems appear, you may need to allow matters to flow more easily. Frustration and annoyance can be countered by directing your attention elsewhere, to where harmony and relaxation reside. In a positive position, these gems can show harmony in relationships; in a difficult cast, they may show areas of friction.

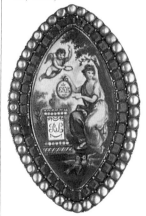

Above Pearls have long been linked with mourning, and were typically used to adorn memorial brooches.

81

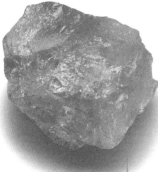

Rose Quartz

Rose quartz is considered to be one of the most powerful stones for emotional healing.

Rose quartz is an uncommon variety of quartz. It occurs primarily in massive, microcrystalline form; only very recently have larger crystals been found in some Brazilian mines. Transparent, gem-quality rose quartz is also rare – most specimens are cloudy. Rose quartz is very brittle and often contains many fractures. Because of its high value, it is used almost exclusively for jewellery and ornamentation. The pink colour is thought to derive from titanium or manganese oxides.

Myth and history

Rose quartz was highly valued in the classical world both for its decorative qualities and its healing properties. The Romans imported rose quartz from mines in Sri Lanka, India, and even Russia. Carved intaglios and cameos, as well as personal seal rings, still exist from this period.

Rose quartz

Colour: pink, rose, peach, violet-pink
Hardness: 7
Composition: SiO_2
Qualities: emotional release, calming
Main chakra: heart

Spiritual and healing properties

Rose quartz is an effective stone for reducing all aggravating or aggressive conditions. It encourages better understanding and increases self-worth. Further, it helps to neutralise the damage caused by poor self-image and a build-up of emotional stress, both of which can prevent effective healing. Placed close to the heart, large pieces of rose quartz can release stress and trauma rapidly. Sometimes this process can cause discomfort, and so care should be taken to balance the release with calming and stabilizing stones.

Suggested Crystal Readings

Rose quartz in centre/First House
Be loving and supportive of those around you.

Rose quartz in southeast/Second House
A lack of self-confidence may be at the root of your current situation.

Rose quartz in east/Third House
Be sensitive when speaking to others.

Rose quartz in north/Fourth House
You need to focus on turning your home into a more loving and caring environment.

Rose quartz in west/Fifth House
Emotional times for new relationships and relationships with children are ahead.

Rose quartz in Sixth House
Be kind to yourself. Being overcritical and a perfectionist is causing you stress and anxiety.

Rose quartz in southwest/Seventh House
Accept those close to you for who and what they are.

Rose quartz in Eighth House
You may be oversensitive to the moods of others, which leaves you feeling tired.

Rose quartz in northeast/Ninth House
Meeting up with friends more often will help boost your confidence.

Rose quartz in south/Tenth House
Be kind and open, but most of all be firm in your dealings with others.

Rose quartz in northwest/Eleventh House
A misunderstanding may have caused problems with friends. Work out your differences.

Rose quartz in Twelfth House
Look closely at how you see yourself. You may find that you need to change your negative impressions.

Personality
Rose Quartz represents a person who is empathic, sympathetic, and supportive of other people's lives. Emotional expression is strong and forthright, with no hidden agendas or manipulation.

Energy
Emotional, loving, sensitive.

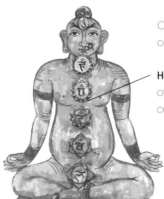

Crystals are placed on the heart chakra

Heart chakra centre of breastbone in centre of chest

83

Divinatory interpretation

Rose quartz is the stone of relationships. It relates to friends, lovers, and those areas of our lives to which we devote a lot of emotional energy. Whatever we feel sustains us is represented by rose quartz. The position in which the stone falls in a reading shows not only where we are strongest, but also where we are the most sensitive.

In a difficult placement, rose quartz may show fissures in self-image and self-confidence. There may be problems with aggression or misunderstandings. In a positive placement, the stone will confirm a situation of support, friendship, emotional well-being, and love.

Above Rough pieces of rose quartz are often just as attractive as rare, translucent, gem-quality specimens.

Right Rose quartz is particularly useful for balancing the energies in a relationship, especially where there is a lack of confidence or trust.

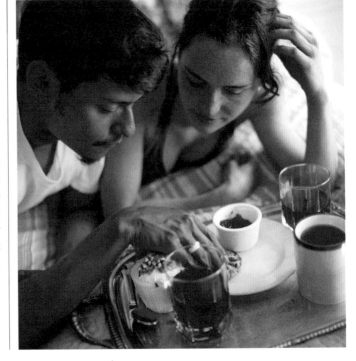

Rubellite in Lepidolite

The harmonious blend of these two minerals can help free us from the influences of the past.

R ubellite is a red variety of tourmaline that often grows in the same environment as lepidolite. Lepidolite, also known as lithium mica, forms deep in the ground under igneous conditions. It grows in small, rough scales, and is commonly found as a massive aggregate with a beautiful purple-pink colour. Like all mica, it has a very reflective surface, so the pink rock shimmers and glistens in its rough form. Lepidolite is a source of the rare metal lithium, which is used in the making of alloys and batteries.

Myth and history

When lepidolite contains the rare element rubidium, it can be used for geological dating. Although relatively soft and fragile, it is often worn as a gemstone, tumbled or polished into a cabochon to show its pearly lustre and deep colour to best advantage.

Rubellite often intergrows with lepidolite, showing as lengths of pink or red tourmaline throughout the rock. As with many other coloured, transparent tourmalines, rubellite has a long history of being cut as a gemstone.

Spiritual and healing properties

Rubellite is a fine balancer for the heart chakra, and can help energise and stabilise the emotions; it is calming in its paler varieties and more stimulating in its darker tones. Rubellite clears away aggression, and helps to introduce more assertiveness where there is too much acceptance and passivity. Pink stones help to balance the creative aspects of the sacral chakra, where deep trauma tends to be stored.

Lepidolite
Colour: grey-pink, purple-grey
Hardness: 2.5–4
Composition:
$K(Li,Al)_3(Si,Al)_4O_{10}(F,OH)_2$ (lithium mica)
Qualities: honest, forgiving
Main chakra: heart, crown

85

Suggested Crystal Readings

Rubellite in lepidolite in centre/First House
You have a need to be seen to be at peace with yourself.

Rubellite in lepidolite in southeast/ Second House
Judging yourself too harshly only damages you – give yourself the praise you deserve.

Rubellite in lepidolite in east/Third House
Ignore any gossip or idle chatter about yourself or about those around you.

Rubellite in lepidolite in north/Fourth House
Deep emotional problems within your family need to be brought to the surface.

Rubellite in lepidolite in west/Fifth House
You will attract love and attention only when you feel that you deserve it.

Rubellite in lepidolite in Sixth House
Make a specific effort to rest and relax to give your body time to heal.

Rubellite in lepidolite in southwest/ Seventh House
It is time to settle disagreements or arguments in close relationships.

Rubellite in lepidolite in Eighth House
Allow resentment about old hurts to be released or dissolved.

Rubellite in lepidolite in northeast/Ninth House
Be careful not to blame others for missed opportunities or spoiled chances.

Rubellite in lepidolite in south/Tenth House
Be aware that in your effort to reach your goals, you may have upset others.

Rubellite in lepidolite in northwest/ Eleventh House
Don't let other people overlook your presence or opinions – stand up and be noticed.

Rubellite in lepidolite in Twelfth House
If you feel like a victim, resolve the issue in another way.

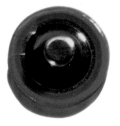

Lepidolite is best known for its ability to reduce stress and soothe the emotions. With its purple and pink colouration, it produces the same calming effect as is achieved when amethyst and rose quartz are paired together. All aspects of self-esteem are strengthened, encouraging honest, open levels of communication.

When found unified as a single stone, rubellite in lepidolite is an ideal combination for clearing emotional debris from the past away from the aura and the heart.

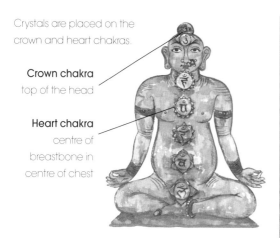

Crystals are placed on the crown and heart chakras.

Crown chakra
top of the head

Heart chakra
centre of breastbone in centre of chest

Personality

Rubellite in lepidolite may suggest someone who is trapped in the past in some way, and cannot forget an event – either positive or traumatic in nature – that happened to them. Alternatively, it may represent someone who deals with history and the passage of time.

Energy

Accepting, reconciliatory.

Divinatory interpretation

Rubellite in lepidolite in a reading shows the influence of the past arising to affect events in the present. In a positive setting, it shows that the questioner is gathering the fruits of positive actions. Relaxation at the end of a long process of creativity is well deserved, and the questioner should sit back and enjoy the results.

When rubellite in lepidolite is surrounded by more difficult energies, it can show that the questioner may be feeling shame or guilt for some real or imagined occurrence. Alternatively, it may show that negativity is being directed at the questioner from those who feel that he or she is to blame for something.

Rubellite in lepidolite can also indicate feuds, grudges, or resentments held over considerable periods of time that sour relationships. The lesson of this blend of stones is that forgiveness and acceptance – together with the negative polarity of blame and resentment – stem from the self. Such emotions are simply a mirroring of our own problems with the world. If we act to release the hurt from ourselves, the process of reconciliation will spontaneously begin.

Facing Page
Lepidolite is an important source of lithium for batteries.

Below Lepidolite can bring clarity to troubled relationships.

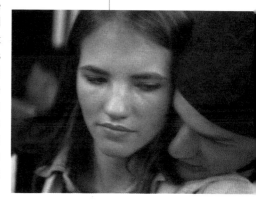

Garnet

Garnet can spark into flame anything that comes into contact with its fiery nature.

Garnet is formed at very high temperatures, from a complex mixture of minerals with similar compositions. Because of this method of formation, garnet has a wider range of colour than any other stone, though the best known and most sought after are the red varieties. Garnets are often found as large granules or clusters within rock, and are roughly ball-shaped, with many facets. They are dense and break easily, though their sharp edges make them ideal as an abrasive material.

Garnet

Colour: red, brown, orange, green
Hardness: 6.5 –7.5
Composition: X_3Y_2 $(SiO_4)_3$ where X and Y are various metals (silicates of bivalent and trivalent elements)
Qualities: energising, accelerating
Main chakra: base

Myth and history

Ragiel's Book of Wings, a thirteenth-century mystical text, says that "The well-formed image of a lion, if engraved on a garnet, will protect and preserve diarrhoeas and health, cure the wearer of all diseases, bring him diarrhoeas, and guard him from all perils in travelling."

The name "garnet" is thought to derive from the Latin word *punica granatum*, meaning pomegranate, because of the resemblance of the seeds to the stone.

Spiritual and healing properties

The particular colour of a garnet specimen will determine its exact effect, but garnet will always work to focus and activate. Red garnets are the best energising stones for the body, speeding up all processes and amplifying the effects of other stones placed

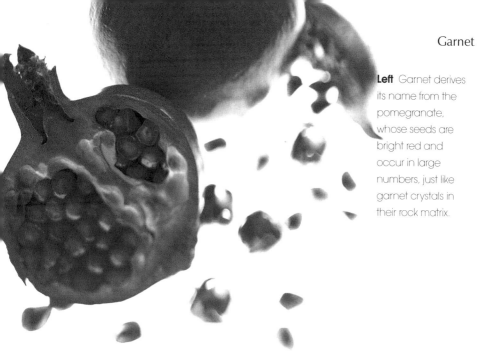

Left Garnet derives its name from the pomegranate, whose seeds are bright red and occur in large numbers, just like garnet crystals in their rock matrix.

nearby. All garnets are useful to get things under way, although it is sometimes better to let other stones continue the work. Any cool, sluggish, watery conditions and states can be balanced by the energy of garnet, which introduces the fire element.

Divinatory interpretation

Garnet is an energiser and motivator; all dull, stagnant situations can be revitalised by its energy. It tends to amplify the strength of other stones – both their positive and difficult qualities – depending on the cast. Positively, garnet will stimulate and activate. Negatively, it will irritate and annoy. It can denote passion, but not necessarily of the long-lasting variety. It can show anger that flares up but quickly dies down again, and can suggest new ideas or creativity that will fizzle out or become distracted if not balanced by other, more grounded, qualities. Like fire, garnet can sustain life and liveliness, or it can cause pain and burning.

Personality

Garnet represents someone who is busy, obsessive, and somewhat impatient. A live wire, this person will always cause a stir wherever he or she goes – sometimes positive, sometimes negative, but never subtle.

Energy

Active, energetic, unfocused.

Suggested Crystal Readings

Garnet in centre/First House
Action is needed now, while energy is still available.

Garnet in southeast/Second House
This is not a good time to make decisions about long-term projects. Wait a few days.

Garnet in east/Third House
The temptation to respond quickly may worsen matters.

Garnet in north/Fourth House
Don't let anything stagnate in your home – deal with matters quickly.

Garnet in west/Fifth House
Be philosophical about short-lived relationships or ideas that might come to nothing.

Garnet in Sixth House
You need to tackle matters with more enthusiasm and energy. You could be prone to mild illness.

Garnet in southwest/Seventh House
People in partnerships are likely to irritate you. Try to ignore this, although it may annoy you.

Garnet in Eighth House
Your own anger or that of others could temporarily distract your attention.

Garnet in northeast/Ninth House
Start to explore new possibilities and new horizons.

Garnet in south/Tenth House
You need to be daring, and to move the situation along quickly in order to achieve what you want.

Garnet in northwest/Eleventh House
Take a chance with a new friend or with new group activities, but do not do so in a serious way.

Garnet in Twelfth House
Look closely at your own habits if you find yourself the target of minor accidents or angry outbursts.

Facing Page Where there is a need for energy, dynamism, and action, a deep red garnet stone will have an immediate stimulating effect.

Crystals are placed on the base chakra.

Base (root) chakra
Base of spine (perineum)

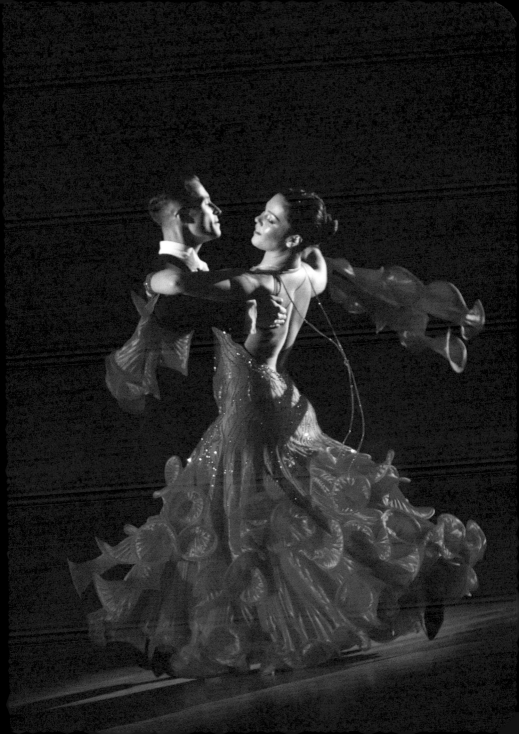

Ruby

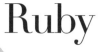

Ruby is traditionally thought of as a stone of the heart and of the sun – both the centre of our being and the centre of our solar system.

Below In the Ayurvedic traditions of India, ruby is the gemstone that holds and amplifies the properties of the sun.

R uby is a variety of the hard mineral corundum. The red colouration is caused by small amounts of chromium. It is a difficult stone to imitate well because the colour changes depending on the angle of view.

Suggested Crystal Readings

Ruby in centre/First House
Make sure to let people know that you are confident and optimistic.

Ruby in southeast/Second House
Be careful with personal finances, but trust that everything will work out.

Ruby in east/Third House
Helpful people surround you, so place your trust in what they offer.

Ruby in north/Fourth House
An infusion of energy and emotion into your home life will help things remain steady.

Ruby in west/Fifth House
You need to be encouraged to take a chance with your own abilities.

Ruby in Sixth House
Confidence at work will carry the situation through for you.

Ruby in southwest/Seventh House
Honesty and openness are needed in all of your relationships.

Ruby in Eighth House
You may be called upon to support someone emotionally or financially, or you may need help yourself.

Ruby in northeast/Ninth House
Keep looking at the positive side of events.

Ruby in south/Tenth House
Sudden changes of plans and direction are unwise. Stick to tried and successful ideas.

Ruby in northwest/Eleventh House
Friends may ask for your support now to help give them the confidence they need.

Ruby in Twelfth House
Quiet periods spent alone are needed to sustain you through this busy time and to help keep your stress levels low.

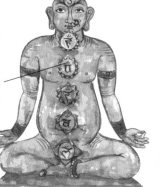

Crystals are placed on the heart chakra.

Heart chakra centre of breastbone in centre of chest

Personality

A ruby personality is open, warm, friendly, and confident. This person is a natural leader who shows responsibility for others, and is honest and trustworthy.

Energy

Encouraging, helpful, sustaining.

Corundum forms characteristic hexagonal, barrel-shaped crystals, and has been collected from riverbank deposits in southeast Asia for thousands of years. Star ruby is a valuable variation in which tiny crystals of rutile inclusions create an asterism – a starlike refraction of light upon the polished surface of the stone. Synthetic rubies are often used in precision tools such as watches and lasers.

Myth and history

In India, the ruby is the most prized of all gemstones, as it is thought to carry the beneficent energy of the sun. Traditionally, large and transparent rubies were uncommon, and thus symbolised wealth and power. Rubies were associated with the energy of inextinguishable flame and of inner radiance, and were thought to confer peace, abundance, wealth, and protection. Actually sewn into the flesh, a ruby was thought to make a soldier invulnerable.

Above Gem-quality ruby has the colour and translucency of drops of blood, making its link to the life force all the more apparent.

Ruby

Colour: red
Hardness: 9
Composition: $Al_2O_3 + Cr$ (corundum)
Qualities: balanced, positive, secure
Main chakra: heart

Spiritual and healing properties

The physical heart and the heart chakra are the centres of the physical and subtle bodies, and have an important effect on every organ and bodily system. The ruby, which acts on all levels of the heart, is thus an important healing stone. If the heart is truly in balance, everything else follows naturally. A sense of harmony, ease, self-confidence, and clarity of mind are engendered, and these qualities naturally enhance our relationships with others. Star ruby emphasises the spiritual levels of the heart, the relationship of the individual to the divine, and an increase in the flow of life energy.

Divinatory interpretation

Ruby will have a positive influence wherever it appears in a reading, and will positively affect the stones that are close by. Ruby is supporting, optimistic, and encouraging. It brings a sense of security to all activity, and will imbue everything with a beneficial life-giving energy. In relationships, ruby shows honesty, openness, and levels of emotional harmony; in work and everyday life, ruby shows contentment and self-confidence. In health matters, ruby may suggest the need to look after the heart, physically or emotionally, especially if situated near other warning stones.

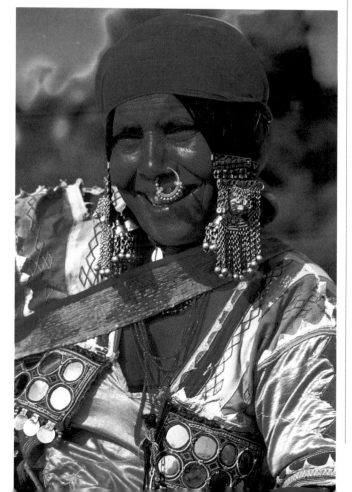

Left Many peoples around the world, particularly from nomadic tribes, wear their wealth in the form of jewellery made from precious metals and adorned with gemstones.

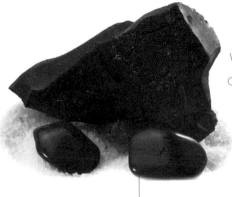

Red Jasper

Within the great variety of colours
and patterns in jasper is the steady,
practical energy of the Earth.

Red jasper forms in veins and slabs from quartz solutions containing hematite, giving it its characteristic brick-red colour. This stone is an opaque, microcrystalline variety of quartz. Often, the patterning and colour variations in each piece have been created by periods of recrystallisation, whereby the rock is fractured and rearranged, usually with other quartz inclusions. Because the structure contains tiny pores, jasper and other quartzes readily take on the colour of the surrounding rock.

Red jasper

Colour: red mixed with other colours
Hardness: 7
Composition: SiO_2 (quartz family)
Qualities: energizing, practical skills
Main chakra: base

Myth and history

The meaning of the name "jasper" is unknown, but it is thought to be traceable back to the word *ashpu*, the Assyrian name for the stone. Jasper is frequently mentioned in the Bible, and is listed as one of the foundations of the Heavenly City described in John's vision in the Book of Revelation.

Jasper was used for ornaments and amulets throughout the ancient world and Middle Ages. The attraction of the stone was that every piece was unique in its colour and markings, yet it could be found in large enough volumes for carving vases, tables, and wall slabs for palaces and churches. Jasper was also popular in the past as a protection against the bites of snakes and other venomous animals, and against the effects of poison.

Suggested Crystal Readings

Red jasper in centre/First House
Keep your feet on the ground regardless of what is going on around you.

Red jasper in southeast/Second House
You need to value your skills more and put them to better use.

Red jasper in east/Third House
Be honest in your communications. Bending the truth will only lead to trouble.

Red jasper in north/Fourth House
Take time to finish off day-to-day jobs at home.

Red jasper in west/Fifth House
Use leisure time to develop the extra skills needed for future endeavours.

Red jasper in Sixth House
Start doing the job at hand – don't question why, just get going.

Red jasper in southwest/Seventh House
Relationships might take more effort than expected. Don't put your partners on pedestals.

Red jasper in Eighth House
Your money should be working for you. Make sure that you are not losing out through careless management.

Red jasper in northeast/Ninth House
Study whichever subjects you want – put your knowledge to practical use.

Red jasper in south/Tenth House
Look at the practicalities of your future plans to see if they are realistic.

Red jasper in northwest/Eleventh House
Be honest with friends and acquaintances and you will reap the benefits.

Red jasper in Twelfth House
Try not to reach for goals that are unattainable. Stick to what you know you can do.

Personality
The person corresponding to jasper is down-to-earth and straightforward, though by no means simple to define. He or she is good at making useful things, and is not interested in vague dreams or flights of imagination.

Energy
Skilful, practical, down-to-earth.

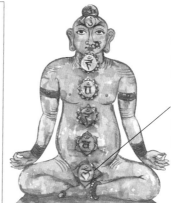

Crystals are placed on the base chakra.

Base (root) chakra
base of spine
(perineum)

97

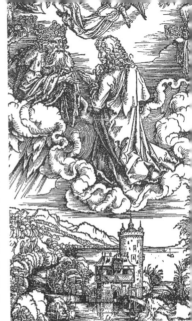

Spiritual and healing properties

Jasper is earthy, solid, and dependable, and focuses energy at the base chakra in a way that is gently grounding. It encourages practicality and down-to-earth realism. With its many colours and patterns, jasper can also help to stimulate psychic faculties, dreams, and visionary skills, though its main focus is always to repair and enhance the physical structures of the body.

Divinatory interpretation

Wherever jasper appears in a reading, it indicates the need to focus on practical, visible outcomes. Do what is necessary – do not waste time and effort on complicated schemes and elaborate strategies. Jasper is an opaque stone, and so everything reflected on its surface appears as it really is. This opacity is a signal to take things at face value – nothing is being hidden from you. Devious actions by others will come to nothing if you act honestly and openly. Jasper will also provide sufficient practical skills to accomplish goals, particularly of a physical or material nature.

Right Many different types of stones, including jasper, were traditionally thought to possess the power to ward off attacks from venomous creatures.

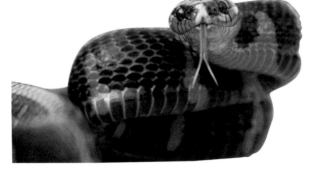

Rhodonite

The deep salmon-pink
colouration of rhodonite
has made it a popular
carving stone.

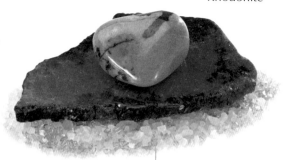

Rhodonite forms in metamorphic rocks such as marble, where there is a high manganese content. It mainly occurs in evenly grained massive form which, together with its colouration, make it ideal as a carving material. Crystals are rare, and are table-top-shaped when they appear. Rhodonite is very often characterised by dark veins of manganese oxides, which increase its value as a gemstone. It is usually translucent, though transparent forms do occur.

Myth and history

Identified only in 1819, rhodonite takes its name from the Greek word *rhodon*, meaning "rose." Sources of quality crystals include Brazil, Finland, Japan, and Mexico. The mineral is often used to make ornamental figures and large objets d'art; it is also used in ceramic glazes and artists' pigments.

Spiritual and healing properties

The colour of rhodonite helps bring balance to the heart chakra, ensuring a realistic and practical approach to the emotions and to emotional responses. The darker colours within the pink hue bring a stabilising and grounding energy that can be useful for alleviating negative states such as confusion and anxiety. The magenta tones boost confidence and motivation.

Rhodonite

Colour: pink, dark pink with veins of black or brown

Hardness: 5.5–6.5

Composition: $CaMn_4(SiO_3)_5$ (silicate of manganese and calcium)

Qualities: empowering, practical, compassionate

Main chakra: heart

Suggested Crystal Readings

Rhodonite in centre/First House
Let others see you as having learned from past mistakes.

Rhodonite in southeast/Second House
Address poor management of personal resources, if security is desired.

Rhodonite in east/Third House
You may need to tone down personal feelings when explaining to others where problems lie.

Rhodonite in north/Fourth House
Look for old emotional patterns that keep recurring and take steps to deal with them.

Rhodonite in west/Fifth House
Indulge yourself in a luxury you seldom have the chance to enjoy.

Rhodonite in Sixth House
Prominent health issues may need a complementary approach – try crystal healing, acupuncture, or shiatsu.

Rhodonite in southwest/Seventh House
Emotional vulnerability in close relationships needs to be examined and understood.

Rhodonite in Eighth House
Take time out to support others who are having difficulties, but only if you can offer them practical suggestions.

Rhodonite in northeast/Ninth House
Tackle new projects or ideas enthusiastically, but stay focused on the practical issues.

Rhodonite in south/Tenth House
Be pleased with yourself for what you have managed to achieve.

Rhodonite in northwest/Eleventh House
Help others to feel confident in themselves and their skills.

Rhodonite in Twelfth House
Be open to the problems of other people, but don't get emotionally involved.

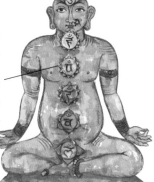

Crystals are placed on the heart chakra.

Heart Chakra
centre of breastbone in centre of chest.

Personality
This crystal is characterised by either a very grounded, passionate, down-to-earth person, or by one who lacks assuredness and self-confidence.

Energy
Practical, motivated, insecure.

Rhodonite is also thought to be useful for those who work with mantras and the subtle qualities of sound, as it increases the practitioner's sensitivity.

Divinatory interpretation

Rhodonite appearing in a reading warns that the questioner must be practical in any emotional decision-making. In other words, don't get carried away with what might be. Focus on the present moment and what is possible and safe to achieve. A failure to be practical now will only add to any confusion or anxiety.

In a positive placement, rhodonite shows that emotional relationships have a firm, solid basis, resting on mutual appreciation and understanding. Where it appears in a placement related directly to the questioner, issues linked to self-esteem and self-confidence need to be addressed. There may be a lack of self-love, or perhaps too much self-confidence. Either extreme will present difficulties in acting appropriately in the situation at hand. In either of these circumstances, balance can be achieved by recognising and removing emotional baggage from the past that is influencing present relationships. A good way forward is to see if there are any repeating patterns occurring in your relationships. Are the same types of personalities involved? Do the same sorts of scenarios keep reappearing? Although breaking a pattern risks letting the unexpected occur, it is the only way forward in a negative cycle.

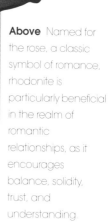

Above Named for the rose, a classic symbol of romance, rhodonite is particularly beneficial in the realm of romantic relationships, as it encourages balance, solidity, trust, and understanding.

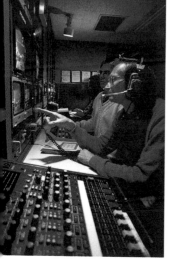

Left Sound, particularly music, has a direct effect upon both the emotions and the heart chakra. Rhodonite can help balance these areas, thereby increasing emotional stability.

101

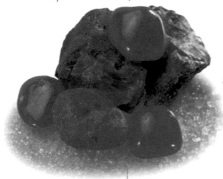

Carnelian

A stone of gentle healing, carnelian
exudes a warmth that is both
soothing and very powerful.

Carnelian is a variety of quartz known as chalcedony. Chalcedony forms in a different manner from rock crystal, in tightly packed layers or rounded aggregates of very fine fibres. It is the pores between these fibres that allow chalcedony to exist in such a variety of colours. Nearly all of these varieties have been given distinct names – carnelian, jasper, chrysoprase, to name a few – and most have a history of decorative use.

Chalcedony crystallises in pockets of rock where silica-rich gel collects. It also forms from the erosion of other minerals, such as serpentine.

Carnelian

Colour: red-orange
Hardness: 7
Composition: SiO_2 (silicon dioxide – chalcedony)
Qualities: healing, soothing, creative
Main chakra: sacral

Right An Egyptian carnelian seal ring from the 2nd millennium BC carved with the seals of Ramses II and Nefertiti.

Myth and history

Found in India, Arabia, and Egypt, carnelian was highly valued as a gemstone in ancient times, particularly the orange variety, known as "sard." It was used to carve early Babylonian cylinders for recording information and for official and personal seals. In ancient Egypt, carnelian was one of the main stones used to make amulets into which were carved extracts from The Book of the Dead. Carnelian is also one of the stones in the High Priest's breastplate mentioned in the Book of Exodus, verse 27. Here it is called odem, and

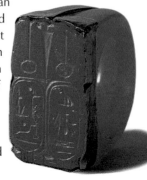

102

Suggested Crystal Readings

Carnelian in centre/First House
Take events as they come. Don't let anything faze or upset you.

Carnelian in southeast/Second House
Now is the time to deal with old emotional pain that has recently surfaced.

Carnelian in east/Third House
Take care to insure that you are completely understood in your communications.

Carnelian in north/Fourth House
You need to take time out to relax at home or away from crowds of people.

Carnelian in west/Fifth House
Put aside time to just enjoy being alive, without the pressures of your world.

Carnelian in Sixth House
If you are having health problems, you may benefit from a visit to a healer.

Carnelian in southwest/Seventh House
Insure good communication so that harsh words or actions in partnerships are clarified and understood.

Carnelian in Eighth House
If financial deals or emotional ties are holding you back, consider releasing them for good.

Carnelian in northeast/Ninth House
Sharing your knowledge will help others to recover from past problems.

Carnelian in south/Tenth House
Creativity and adaptability are needed for success and its enjoyment.

Carnelian in northwest/Eleventh House
Time spent repairing friendships that have been recently bruised will help all concerned.

Carnelian in Twelfth House
Pay attention to personal requirements and look for ways to meet your needs.

Personality
Carnelian represents a warm, friendly, caring, and sympathetic person who has experienced much in life. This person is also creative, nurturing, sensual, and sensitive.

Energy
Healing, creative, sympathetic.

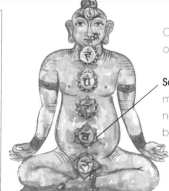

Crystals are placed on the sacral chakra.

Sacral chakra
midway between navel and pubic bone.

103

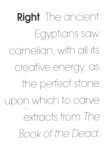

is associated with the tribe of Reuben. In classical Greece and Rome, carnelian was one of the most popular materials for carving magical amulets.

Today, the finest carnelian, which has a red-orange colour, comes from the vicinity of Bombay, India.

Spiritual and healing properties

As a healing stone, carnelian is gently activating and warming, and will encourage the natural healing abilities of the body. This is partly because it energises the sacral chakra, where stress and trauma tends to become lodged. Carnelian helps to gently release these imbalances, even if they have been present for many years. Orange is one of the best colours to use where shock, or an accident or illness have occurred. Where there is rigidity, stiffness, or inflammation, carnelian can help to restore the correct energy flow.

Right The ancient Egyptians saw carnelian, with all its creative energy, as the perfect stone upon which to carve extracts from *The Book of the Dead.*

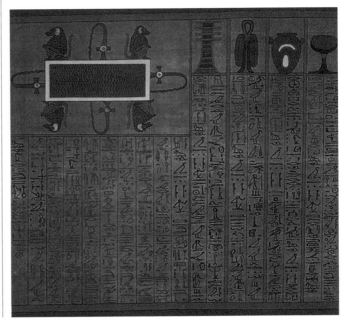

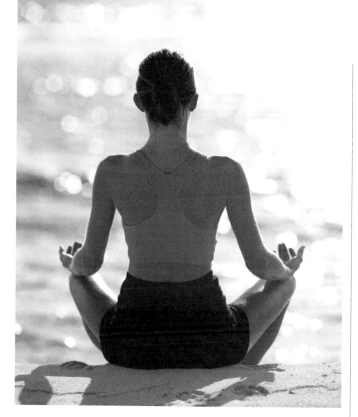

Divinatory interpretation

In a positive placement, carnelian indicates a great deal of creative energy. Love of life, happiness, enjoyment, and harmony with those around you are all suggested by this stone. Carnelian also represents the energy of movement and the flexibility of "going with the flow." It suggests that you should work with that which presents itself to you, rather than forging ahead in search of a distant goal. Both success and an increase in positive energies are favoured by this stone.

In a difficult position, carnelian may warn that flexibility should be encouraged, or you may find yourself suffering from the negative associations of this stone, including stress, illness, inertia, and an inability to progress. Deep pain and old wounds may also need attention before they create further problems.

Copper

Copper, which forms natural nuggets and treelike shapes, was the first metal to be worked by humankind.

Copper

Colour: orange-red with green oxides, metallic

Hardness: 2.5–3

Composition: Cu (elemental copper)

Qualities: harmonising, flowing, calming

Main chakra: base, sacral, solar plexus, heart

Right Copper bracelets are an effective way to reduce inflammation and pain. They can also help ease the effects of difficult planetary positions, such as emotional swings and mental upset.

C opper is formed from the alteration of copper-bearing solutions and other minerals. Native copper, the natural crystals or nuggets, is formed in zones where other copper ores are located. Copper ores, which are usually a strong green colour, are very common. The metal has a low melting point and can be easily worked due to its softness. Like most elemental metals, copper is a good conductor of electricity, and is in great demand for electrical wiring.

Myth and history

Copper's name derives from the Roman words *Cyprium aes*, meaning "metal from Cyprus," where the Romans found plentiful supplies. Copper was the first metal to be used by humankind simply because, unlike most other metals, it was found in pure, soft, workable nuggets.

About 8,000 years ago, copper was beaten into simple tools. At some point it began to be melted, and was then added to tin ore to make bronze, a much stronger alloy. By about 4000 BC bronze had become the main material for weapons, tools, and ornaments. Later, copper became a major source of wealth from trade, and created important links among far-flung cultures.

Suggested Crystal Readings

Copper in centre/First House
You need to show others that you can cope with anything and are willing to start again.

Copper in southeast/Second House
You may be creating your own difficulties by maintaining inappropriate or rigid views.

Copper in east/Third House
Keep all communication lines open and delay any decisions until you have all the information you need.

Copper in north/Fourth House
Insure that any emotional tension with family members is released before it has the chance to become established.

Copper in west/Fifth House
Leisure activities and romance may seem to be at a standstill. Have patience.

Copper in Sixth House
Consider taking advice from others with respect to health or work situations.

Copper in southwest/Seventh House
Seeing another person's viewpoint will avoid unnecessary conflict with those dear to you.

Copper in Eighth House
Delays in money matters could cause frustration. Just accept situations that you cannot alter.

Copper in northeast/Ninth House
Examine what may be stopping you from exploring matters further.

Copper in south/Tenth House
If you wish to get things moving along, you must pay more attention to the situation in hand.

Copper in northwest/Eleventh House
Friends and colleagues may need you to act as a diplomat to settle some disagreements.

Copper in Twelfth House
You need time alone to integrate and absorb all that is happening.

Crystals are placed on the heart, solar plexus, sacral, and base chakras.

Solar plexus chakra midway between navel and base of ribs

Base (root) chakra base of spine (perineum)

Heart chakra centre of breastbone in centre of chest

Sacral chakra midway between navel and pubic bone

107

Right In ancient
Roman mythology,
copper was
associated magically
with Venus, both the
planet and the
goddess. In ancient
Greek mythology,
Cyprus, where
copper is abundant,
is said to be the
birthplace of the
goddess Aphrodite
(the Greek name for
Venus), whose name
means "of the foam."

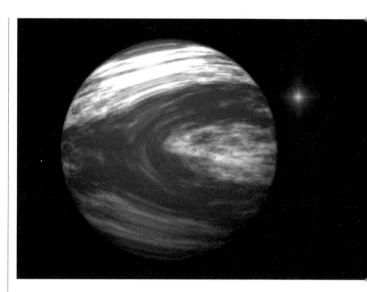

Personality

The copper person is a mediator,
and is able to make positive
suggestions in any situation.
Creative, practical, and flexible,
he or she may appear to be all
things to all people.

Energy

Flexible, mediator, integrated.

Spiritual and healing properties

Copper is often used to reduce the pain and
inflammation of arthritis and rheumatism. It is
not only an excellent conductor of electricity, but
it also helps the flow of many types of energy
throughout the body. Nervous system and
brain functions are strengthened, and there can
be a release of frustration, tension, and
nervous energy.

Divinatory interpretation

Copper will smooth and integrate all energies
that are found around it. If there is potential for
conflict, copper will ease the aggression. If there is resistance or
a blockage preventing movement, copper will help the energy to
flow constructively once more. It will also help all communications
and improve emotional situations.

Copper reminds us to remain open to negotiation, to be
willing to accept new input, and not to become irritated by the
behaviour of others.

Pyrite

Pyrite (or iron pyrites) is commonly known as "fool's gold." For those who know its secrets, it can point the way to finding real gold.

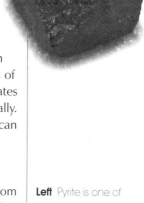

Pyrite is formed when water comes into contact with extremely hot rocks. It usually occurs in granular or massive form, but sometimes crystals of striking cubic appearance are formed. Pyrite creates sulphuric acid as it decomposes, which is exploited industrially. It is also used in paints and polishes. Bits of copper and gold can sometimes occur within pyrites.

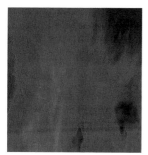

Myth and history

The name of this stone comes from the Greek word *pyr*, meaning fire. When struck or broken, pyrite gives off sparks, and thus it was used in ancient times as a fire-making tool – the ancient precursor to sulphur-dipped matches. Because it shines like the sun and makes fire, we can guess that pyrite must have been a powerful spiritual artefact. The most important spirit for protection and warmth, the perception of fire living within a stone would certainly have made a great impression on our ancestors.

In many ancient civilizations, pyrite was used as a healing amulet, as it was thought to prevent "blood decay." In the civilizations of Central and South America, the Aztecs and Incas cut and polished slabs of pyrite into convex mirrors, many of which were placed in tombs.

Left Pyrite is one of the few common minerals capable of creating fire. Flint and quartz will spark if struck strongly, but pyrite, being softer, is much easier to use.

Pyrite

Colour: metallic yellow
Hardness: 6.5
Composition: FeS_2 (iron sulfide)
Qualities: cleansing, clearing
Main chakra: solar plexus

Suggested Crystal Readings

Pyrite in centre/First House
You may not appear to others as you hope to.

Pyrite in southeast/Second House
It is time to indulge yourself in order to relieve current pressures.

Pyrite in east/Third House
Others could easily misunderstand your intentions, so be cautious.

Pyrite in north/Fourth House
Consider spring cleaning or space clearing at home or in any other personal space.

Pyrite in west/Fifth House
Set aside quiet time to escape into imagined worlds created by yourself.

Pyrite in Sixth House
Clutter and garbage of all kinds – both physical and mental – must be thrown out if you wish to clarify present issues.

Pyrite in southwest/Seventh House
Concerns within relationships and partnerships need to be smoothed over.

Pyrite in Eighth House
Be cautious in any financial dealings; check the details and any advice given.

Pyrite in northeast/Ninth House
Rely on your own experience rather than on those who would impress you with their expertise and knowledge.

Pyrite in south/Tenth House
Reexamine the various jobs you are doing at the moment and cut out those that do not support you.

Pyrite in northwest/Eleventh House
Friends need your compassion and understanding.

Pyrite in Twelfth House
Take time out to reflect on everything that is happening right now.

Crystals are placed on the solar plexus chakra.

Solar plexus chakra
midway between navel and base of ribs

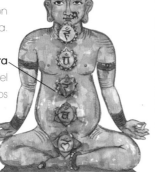

Personality
The pyrite personality is usually difficult to get to know. He or she may be a braggart or simply a dreamer. Shattering the illusion might produce a quick, fiery response.

Energy
Soothing, cleansing, deceptive.

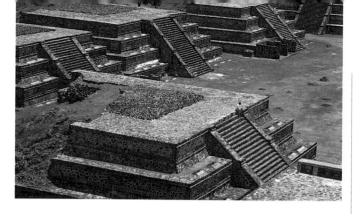

Left The association of pyrite with the sun and fire made it an important material in many ancient cultures. It was particularly valued by Central American civilizations, which tended to focus their ritual worship on the sun and the stars.

Spiritual and healing properties

Pyrite is a combination of iron and sulphur, two important elements for maintaining the physical health of the body. Iron is an essential ingredient of the blood, without which absorption of oxygen into cells becomes impossible. Sulphur is a constituent of amino acids and proteins – the smell of burning hair is primarily sulphur.

Pyrite also helps to regulate the digestive system. Through gentle cleansing action, it is a detoxifying agent that helps protect from pollution and negative forms of energy. Anxiety, frustration, and depression can all be eased using pyrite.

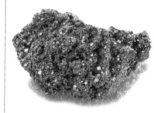

Divination interpretation

The shining, mirrorlike surface of pyrite can reveal what is around it, yet can itself be deceptive. What appears to be golden may in fact be something completely different. Thus, when pyrite appears in a cast, be cautious of appearances. Things are definitely not what they seem, although this deception may not be conscious or malicious.

The nature of some things is to reflect what is around them – our reactions to this reflection often reveal more about ourselves than does the mirror itself. When pyrite appears in a reading, we should ask ourselves what is being mirrored back to us that we find uncomfortable. The lesson of pyrite is to act with awareness – not to simply react to what happens to us. Clear out the debris that clutters your life and prevents you from reflecting your true brightness. In a positive position, pyrite can show itself as an initiator, bringing a spark of inspiration or a sudden clarity of insight. But again, such a spark needs to be carefully examined for its true meaning and value.

Above Pyrite is so common in the Earth's crust that it is found in almost every possible environment, hence its vast number of forms and varieties.

111

Tiger's Eye

Tiger's eye is a striking stone with a lively play of different colours. It is a form of quartz in which the original fibres of asbestos or crocodilite have been replaced by parallel quartz bands.

Tiger's eye has graded bands of yellow and golden brown in various shades. Passing through these bands are parallel silky fibres that have a wonderful sheen as they catch and reflect the light. The orange and yellow tones are created by iron inclusions which, if they come into contact with heat, will turn to the deep red colour of hematite.

Tiger's eye

Colour: yellow to brown, with occasional bands of red and blue
Hardness: 7
Composition: SiO_2 (silicon dioxide)
Qualities: grounding, confidence-building
Main chakra: base, sacral, solar plexus

Myth and history

Tiger's eye is an attractive stone that is usually cut as a "cabochon," a smooth, rounded dome that enhances its natural lustre. Original sources were India and Burma; South Africa and Australia are now important sources as well.

A blue variety of tiger's eye known as hawk's eye or falcon's eye – in which less iron is present in the quartz fibres – also exists. In the valuable cat's-eye stones, light reflects from minute fibres within the transparent crystal in a bright line. Tiger's eye is similar in appearance to these stones but, being opaque, is less valuable.

Spiritual and healing properties

Because of its range of colours, tiger's eye is an excellent stone to balance all three lower chakras: base, sacral, and solar plexus.

Suggested Crystal Readings

Tiger's eye in centre/First House
Be open to working with others, especially those offering practical help.

Tiger's eye in southeast/Second House
Don't rely on your own resources alone to help you in this situation.

Tiger's eye in east/Third House
Talk to others about your ideas. Consider their opinions before you do anything.

Tiger's eye in north/Fourth House
It's time to ask older, more experienced family members for advice and guidance.

Tiger's eye in west/Fifth House
You need to take some risks if you want to succeed.

Tiger's eye in Sixth House
What is needed now is a methodical and steady approach to work, with no sudden changes.

Tiger's eye in southwest/Seventh House
Partnerships and relationships may need extra loving care and attention at the moment.

Tiger's eye in Eighth House
Be cautious where corporate finance is concerned, or where other people have control over your money.

Tiger's eye in northeast/Ninth House
At present there is a possibility for study or travel with friends. Long journeys connected with celebrations may lie ahead.

Tiger's eye in south/Tenth House
Look at the plans you have made for the future and check that you haven't left anything out.

Tiger's eye in northwest/Eleventh House
See if you can involve yourself in a group that shares your goals.

Tiger's eye in Twelfth House
It would be helpful to take part in group activities in which you can forget all the pressures you are under for a while.

Crystals are placed on the solar plexus, sacral, and base chakras.

Solar plexus chakra midway between navel and base of ribs

Sacral chakra midway between navel and pubic bone

Base (root) chakra base of spine (perineum)

113

Right Cat's eye stones can occur in several different types of mineral, where inclusions create a line of light. The qualities of large cats such as the tiger and the leopard suggest that such stones confer stealth, strength, nobility, and grace to the wearer.

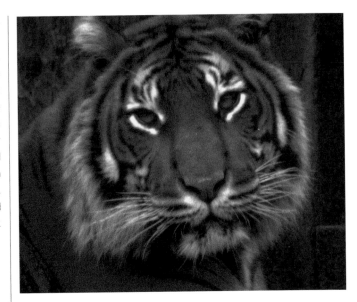

With its fibrous striations, it is able to balance the flow of energy between these centres, thus encouraging confidence, practicality, and an ability to feel at home in the world. Tiger's eye is gently grounding, but the scintillating play of light suggests lightness of touch and an appreciation of joy and beauty, as well as the ability to receive intuitive flashes of information.

Personality

Tiger's eye suggests a warm, sociable, practical person with a good sense of humour. This person may need to always be around people in order to feel comfortable.

Energy

Sociable, practical, group-oriented.

Divinatory interpretation

Tiger's eye has a positive, helpful energy bringing confidence and a practical ability to achieve success. It indicates the need to take a practical, down-to-earth approach to problems or issues. Start with fundamentals and with what you know, and work slowly and methodically from there. Tiger's eye definitely suggests that you shouldn't try to go it alone. We all need help and advice from others, and this stone implies that now is the time to work in groups toward a common objective.

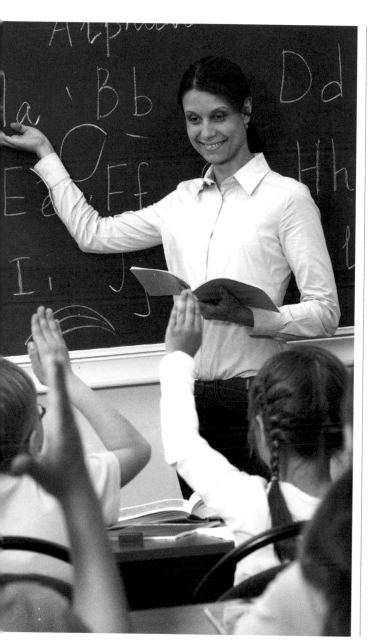

Amber

Amber is thought to carry the
energy of warm sunlight within its
translucent depths.

Below Some classical
philosophers believed
amber to be fossilised
tree resin.

Amber reflects the
very beginnings of
the planet Earth, for
it is the fossilised
resin that dripped from the pine
trees of the forests that grew in the Tertiary Period, over 50
million years ago. Damaged trees leaked resins that fell to the
forest floor and were then covered by deep sediments of sands

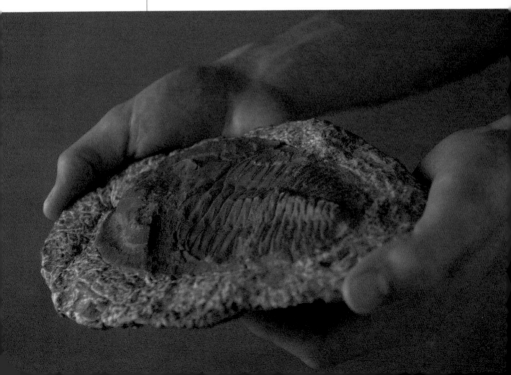

and gravel. After millions of years, erosion washed the amber nodules down to the sea, where they eventually washed upon coastlines.

Myth and history

Amber is found in various parts of the world, including Germany, Canada, and the USA, but the Baltic Sea coasts are its most famous source.

Because it is light and easily worked, amber has been a valuable jewel for thousands of years. Although most amber is cloudy, this cloudiness often clears with gentle heat. Classical poets described amber as the tears of gods, or as the essence of the rays of the setting sun washed up on the sea shore. Amber was also prized in the Roman Empire. The Emperor Nero even mounted an expedition to the Baltic coast to gather his own supplies. In many ancient civilizations, amulets and medicines were commonly made with amber, as it dissolves readily in alcohol.

Spiritual and healing properties

Amber is known as having electrical properties – static electricity is generated when a piece is rubbed. It is thus no surprise that it benefits the electrical systems of the body. Amber can improve the functions of the brain and nervous system, release anxiety, and increase clarity of mind. It is a stimulating compound, but some may find that wearing it for longer than an hour creates irritation or overactivity. It can also be useful for detoxification, and can alleviate depression.

Amber	
Colour:	yellow, yellow-red, red, green
Hardness:	2–2.5
Composition:	complex hydrocarbons (fossil resin)
Qualities:	warming, stimulating
Main chakra:	solar plexus

Below Amber has long been a favoured material for making beads. Worked amber beads have been found in Stone Age burial sites in Scandanavia and Britain.

Suggested Crystal Readings

Amber in centre/First House
An atmosphere of enthusiasm and boundless energy is needed to bring order to the situation.

Amber in southeast/Second House
A renewed drive to cope with personal finances and pull your life together.

Amber in east/Third House
There may be too much talking and not enough listening to other people.

Amber in north/Fourth House
Right now is a busy time at home. A lot of things are happening at once.

Amber in west/Fifth House
You have a myriad of ideas for projects – keep a note of each one so you can review them in quieter times.

Amber in Sixth House
Nervousness and restlessness for long periods of time can cause health problems. Learn to relax.

Amber in southwest/Seventh House
Over-intellectualising can lead to disagreements when emotions are not considered.

Amber in Eighth House
The current rapid pace of events may cause you stress, or may leave you feeling full of energy.

Amber in northeast/Ninth House
Don't take the first opportunity that presents itself. Think things through before committing to anything.

Amber in south/Tenth House
Your energy needs to be focused more carefully – you may have too many projects going on at once.

Amber in northwest/Eleventh House
You have many events to attend and people to meet.

Amber in Twelfth House
Sleep may be temporarily shallow.

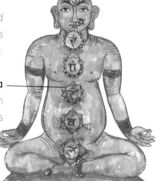

Crystals are placed on the solar plexus chakra.

Solar plexus chakra midway between navel and base of ribs

Personality
Amber personalities are always on the go. They are intelligent and aware, but often find it difficult to sit still or relax. They have a tendency to work too hard and they worry a lot.

Energy
Enlivening, stimulating, electric.

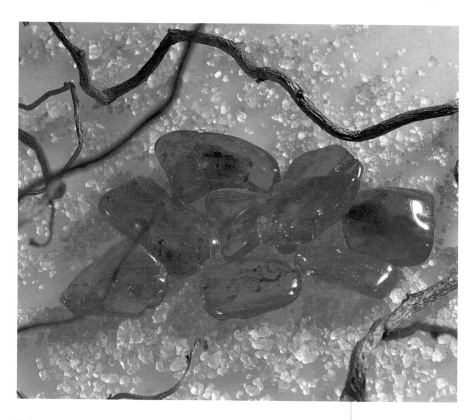

Divinatory interpretation

Amber inserts a certain degree of nervous energy into its surroundings. If found in a placement where other indicators show restriction, stagnancy, and doubt, it acts as a stimulus to get things moving. In a positive or already balanced placement, its presence signals that the questioner needs to take care that things don't get overexcited and frenetic. Amber is like a gemstone caffeine – too much will create chaos, bad temper, and arguments. As long as this excess energy can be used, however, problems will not usually arise.

Where amber appears, watch for skills being underused, for emotions being repressed, and for unalleviated anxieties and tensions.

Above Amber is the energy of trees captured in a stable form, then fossilised for millions of years. This gives amber the ability to generate an extraordinary amount of energy.

119

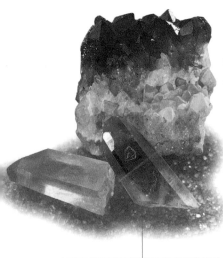

Citrine

Citrine is a transparent yellow variety of quartz crystal that is valued as much for its warm colour as for its rarity.

C itrine occurs naturally where quartz recrystallises with iron inclusions. It can vary in tone from a deep brown-orange to a pale lemon colour.

Citrine

Colour: yellow, golden brown, orange-brown
Hardness: 7
Composition: SiO_2 (quartz)
Qualities: uplifting, warming, confident
Main chakra: solar plexus

Myth and history

Because of its rarity and delicacy of colour, citrine has long been a valuable gemstone. The pale varieties can resemble other precious stones such as heliodor (yellow beryl), chrysoberyl, and some varieties of topaz. During the Middle Ages, citrine was thought to carry the energy of the sun's rays, and thus it was used as a remedy for people whose energy and moods became depressed during the long winter months or during overcast weather.

Right Natural yellow citrine is rare, and so most commercial stones, such as those used for jewellery making, are actually heat-treated amethysts.

Spiritual and healing properties

Citrine's wide range of colours enables it to help balance many different areas of the physical and subtle bodies. The deep orange-brown varieties help to energise the base chakra, and have a gentle grounding effect. Orange-yellow stones work well at the sacral chakra, helping the body to release stress and tension and enjoy life more. Most effective is yellow citrine, which acts at the solar

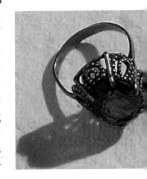

Suggested Crystal Readings

Citrine in centre/First House
An image of confidence will help all situations at this time.

Citrine in southeast/Second House
Take comfort in steady routines that are supportive of present needs.

Citrine in east/Third House
Be clear about all types of communication, even if you have to repeat yourself.

Citrine in north/Fourth House
The roots of the issue are sound and settled, and will provide plenty of security.

Citrine in west/Fifth House
You need to set aside time to relax and have some fun.

Citrine in Sixth House
Look on the bright side of current events to give you the lift you need.

Citrine in southwest/Seventh House
Comfort and kind words from partners will help dissolve anxieties.

Citrine in Eighth House
People with deep concerns find you easy to talk to, but don't become too involved in their problems.

Citrine in northeast/Ninth House
Your thoughts on the larger situation are correct, so trust your intuition.

Citrine in south/Tenth House
The issue can be confidently pushed farther along its path, as long as you consider the well-being of others.

Citrine in northwest/Eleventh House
Quiet times with friends will boost your confidence and calm worries.

Citrine in Twelfth House
Dreams and insights will confirm your present direction.

Personality
The citrine personality is happy, confident, and sunny. These people have a practical side, but they also like to explore the subtle realms of mind and spirit.

Energy
Comforting, uplifting, happy.

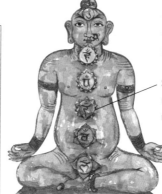

Crystals are placed on the solar plexus chakra.

Solar plexus chakra midway between navel and base of ribs

plexus, balancing the digestive and nervous systems and bringing clarity and focus to the mind. It is gently expansive, relaxing, and comforting, increasing self-confidence and personal power. The golden tones within the crystal also relate to the spiritual energies above the crown of the head, bringing higher levels of wisdom and knowledge. As a grounding stone, citrine helps integrate these levels of intuition into everyday life.

Divinatory interpretation

Citrine brings confidence, the energy to succeed, and a clarity of mind and purpose. It will always help to bring together different energies, particularly if there is a conflict between desire and reality, between an idealist and a pragmatist, or between relaxation and action.

In situations that lack clarity, citrine will bring in the light of the sun to illuminate the problems in such a way as to allow them to be seen for what they are. Citrine requires that thoughts precede actions; thinking the situation through will bring both understanding and the information needed to succeed. Ignoring this stage of the process will likely cause anxiety and confusion.

In a difficult placement, citrine may counsel caution. It can also advise to take things step by step, ensuring that the foundation beneath each step is solid before continuing.

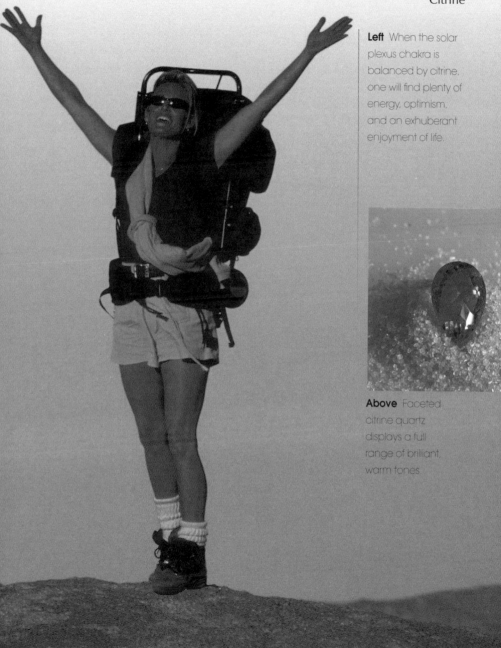

Left When the solar plexus chakra is balanced by citrine, one will find plenty of energy, optimism, and an exhuberant enjoyment of life.

Above Faceted citrine quartz displays a full range of brilliant, warm tones.

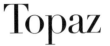

Topaz

Topaz is a very valuable mineral that has been used in jewellery for thousands of years. The most prized varieties are imperial topaz – a rich orange colour – and sherry topaz – a pale yellow colour. Blue topaz bears a strong resemblance to aquamarine.

Topaz

Colour: golden yellow, pink, blue, clear
Hardness: 8
Composition: $Al_2F_2SiO_4$ (aluminum fluorosilicate)
Qualities: energy balancing, stabilizing
Main chakra: solar plexus

Facing Page In the Ayurvedic tradition, topaz comes under the influence of the planet and god Jupiter. Also known as Brihaspati, this deity is the teacher of the gods themselves.

Clear topaz is the most common topaz variety, and has the brilliance of diamond. Colour in this stone is caused by small amounts of various metals in the atomic lattice. Crystals are usually four-sided columns with pyramidal or flat endings. One characteristic of topaz is the vertical striations along the prism faces.

Topaz is sensitive to heat, which will often change the colour of the stone. It is hard but brittle, and can fracture easily. Although popular as a gemstone, topaz is less exclusive than other crystals due to its abundance.

Myth and history

"The figure of a falcon, if on a topaz, helps to acquire the goodwill of kings, princes, and magnates," says a thirteenth-century mystical treatise on gemstone designs.

Some believe the name "topaz" derives from the old name Topazos (now called Zebirgit), an island in the Red Sea on which the Romans discovered a fine source of yellow-green olivine, to which they gave the name topazus. They also used this name for many other yellow gemstones. In fact, old legends which speak of topaz may actually be referring to other yellow gemstones, such as yellow beryl or sapphire, as only recently

Suggested Crystal Readings

Topaz in centre/First House
Be aware that you may appear to be demanding and authoritative to others.

Topaz in southeast/Second House
You need to take charge of your own resources and use them for your own needs.

Topaz in east/Third House
Don't be surprised if others ignore your advice – or if you wind up ignoring theirs.

Topaz in north/Fourth House
Recognise other people's needs when they are visiting you in your home, especially if you want them to stay.

Topaz in west/Fifth House
Your creative skills must be seen to be appreciated. Find ways of expressing them.

Topaz in Sixth House
You work well on your own, but don't be too proud to ask for help if you need it.

Topaz in southwest/Seventh House
Your dominant role in relationships can eclipse your partners' needs and abilities.

Topaz in Eighth House
Don't be pushed around by those who think that they know best, but do listen to what they have to say.

Topaz in northeast/Ninth House
The depth of your knowledge is evident, so don't be boastful when telling others.

Topaz in south/Tenth House
Go for it! This is the ideal time to do what you want and go where you want.

Topaz in northwest/Eleventh House
Social gatherings are a must at this time. Allow others to play a part in the planning and preparation.

Topaz in Twelfth House
Recharge your batteries in situations where someone else is providing you with your practical needs.

have instruments been available to distinguish between these stones. Others believe that the name topaz derives from the Sanskrit word tapas, meaning fire or heat. Topaz is one of the most important of the nine gemstones of Ayurveda, representing the planet Jupiter.

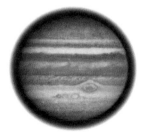

Spiritual and healing properties
Topaz is useful for directing and focusing energy; the stone's parallel striations and natural brilliance help this process. It also cleanses negativity from the emotions, bringing stability and balance. The energies within the self are better organised,

Personality

Topaz has a self-assurance that can be supportive or annoying, depending on how the personality is displayed. A natural leader or a manipulative schemer, this person will always find his or her way into top positions.

Energy

Regal, leader, delegator.

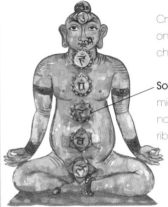

Crystals are placed on the solar plexus chakra.

Solar plexus chakra midway between navel and base of ribs

creating confidence. The solar-plexus chakra – which relates to the maintenance of personal energy levels – is also stimulated by this gemstone. Yellow and golden topaz work well with the crown chakra, increasing peace and harmony, whereas the blue variety can release blockages of communication and expression.

Below The falcon embodies clarity and power, thus making it a fitting image for engraving upon a topaz gemstone.

Divinatory interpretation

In a reading, topaz encourages personal power and leadership. In a positive placement, it can show that now is the time to take the lead, and to gather others around you who can help you in your situation. In this scenario, it is important not to try to do everything yourself – learn to delegate and to trust the qualifications of others. A leader also needs to learn the most effective ways of encouraging others to want to follow his or her suggestions.

In a negative position, topaz suggests that you shouldn't be so domineering and bossy. Give those around you more space. Perhaps you expect to be the centre of attention a little too often. Be aware that other people have needs and priorities too, and that you may not be included in these all of the time.

Topaz teaches us to watch how our energy moves out into the world. Are we being too selfish, narrow-minded, or demanding? Are we relying too much on others, fearful of our own ability to take control of the events that are occurring in our lives?

Rutilated Quartz

Rutilated quartz is a combination of
rock crystal intergrown with crystals
of titanium dioxide called rutile.

I n the modern world, rutile is a valuable
material. Its titanium content is used to make
a corrosion- and heat-resistant ore for use in the steel
industry, as well as light, strong alloys for constructing
aircraft. Rutile forms long, thin, needlelike crystals of golden-
brown or red-brown, and is a common inclusion in quartz veins.

Myth and history

Rutilated quartz is well known in the Alps, where clear quartz can
be found shot through with fine golden threads. Also known as
sagenite or saginitic quartz, rutilated quartz was once a popular
gemstone for a fashion of rings and necklaces known as "hair
of Venus" or "arrows of love." The fine golden
threads bear an uncanny resemblance to locks of
golden hair, which appear to be trapped forever
in the crystal.

Spiritual and healing properties

Rutilated quartz can be of great benefit to
damaged tissue. The interwoven and crossed
patterns of rutile within the quartz stimulate the
repair of wounds by encouraging a multilevel
flow of energy. The stone can also be effective
at restoring normal energy to over- or underactive areas of the
body, the thin golden needles of rutile resembling the complex
interdependence and communication among the systems of
the body. The nervous system and all brain functions are also
stimulated by rutilated quartz.

Rutilated quartz

Colour: transparent or smoky,
with gold or brown inclusions
Hardness: 6–6.5
Composition: SiO_2 + TiO_2 (silicon
dioxide with titanium dioxide)
Qualities: energizing,
regenerating
Main chakra: all

127

Suggested Crystal Readings

Rutilated quartz in centre/First House
An appearance of being focused on the issue or situation will help.

Rutilated quartz in southeast/Second House
Personal finances need to be consolidated and simplified.

Rutilated quartz in east/Third House
Confusing communications are creating problems – find out the truth.

Rutilated quartz in north/Fourth House
Get together with family or close friends for additional security.

Rutilated quartz in west/Fifth House
This is not a good time to take risks or follow whims. Act only when you are confident of the outcome.

Rutilated quartz in Sixth House
Busy times with lots of loose ends can create dissatisfaction. Relax into the situation.

Rutilated quartz in southwest/Seventh House
In the context of relationships, look at the partnership as a whole and not at current frustrations.

Rutilated quartz in Eighth House
Too many demands on your time and money are causing confusion and lack of energy.

Rutilated quartz in northeast/Ninth House
Reduce the distractions of too many ideas and opportunities before making any decisions.

Rutilated quartz in south/Tenth House
This is the right time to consolidate your present position. Pull in others for support where necessary.

Rutilated quartz in northwest/Eleventh House
Working as a group will help you achieve what you cannot manage alone.

Rutilated quartz in Twelfth House
Scattered thoughts and ideas need to be channeled into a single direction.

Crystals are placed on all of the chakras.

Heart chakra centre of breastbone in centre of chest

Sacral chakra midway between navel and pubic bone

Crown chakra top of the head

Brow chakra centre of forehead

Throat chakra neck

Solar plexus chakra midway between navel and base of ribs

Base (root) chakra base of spine (perineum)

128

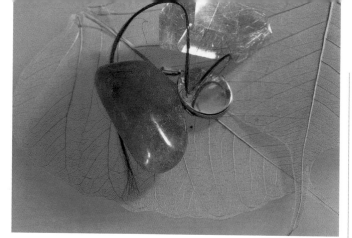

Left One of the most striking varieties of quartz, rutilated quartz resembles blades of grass or hair trapped in crystal.

Divinatory interpretation

Rutilated quartz can show a complex, busy situation where it is necessary to understand and combine many different activities in order to get what you want. In a positive placement, rutilated quartz shows that circumstances are coming together, and that all the energies in a situation are beginning to pull in the same direction. Previously puzzling factors start to make sense, pieces fit into place, and a new coherence emerges.

In a negative placement, this stone may show a failure to integrate all the strands in your life and point them in a uniform direction. This state of affairs can indicate confusion or frustration, with too much going on at once. In these situations, rutilated quartz teaches that it is necessary to focus on the beauty of the whole, rather than trying to isolate and follow each single thread.

In certain placements, this stone may indicate that groups should pull together, or that the individual needs to seek the help of others.

Personality

The rutilated quartz personality has many irons in the fire, and is always busy with different ideas or projects. Poets, inventors, healers, group coordinators, and facilitators fit this stone's energy signature.

Energy

Consolidating, able to work with others.

Left All of the electrically controlled systems of the body benefit from the infusion of energy that rutilated quartz brings.

129

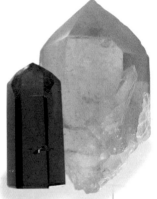

Smoky Quartz

Smoky quartz is a stone of quietness. It contains within its hidden interior the seeds of change and of new beginnings, and the potential for creativity.

Below Smoky quartz encourages the mind to become still and contemplative. New ideas and solutions can suddenly cross the quiet mind.

Smoky quartz has a characteristic smoky brown or grey transparency. The depth of colour can be slight or almost black, and is caused when clear quartz has been exposed to natural sources of radiation – either from within the Earth or from ultraviolet wavelengths. Occasionally, manganese impurities are present. Smoky quartz is usually found in mountainous areas.

Myth and history

The Romans were well-aquainted with this stone; the dark, almost opaque black variety is called "morion" after the Latin name for it. A golden-brown variety of smoky quartz is found in

Suggested Crystal Readings

Smoky quartz in centre/First House
Clarity is needed in the way in which a situation or person is being portrayed.

Smoky quartz in southeast/Second House
Reexamine your thoughts on projects that have not yet begun. Do they need changing?

Smoky quartz in east/Third House
It may be better to remain quiet or restrained.

Smoky quartz in north/Fourth House
Spend time at home thinking about the entire situation.

Smoky quartz in west/Fifth House
Focus on how you are actually going to begin or initiate plans.

Smoky quartz in Sixth House
Changes may be needed in the way you work.

Smoky quartz in southwest/Seventh House
Adjustments in relationships are likely.

Smoky quartz in Eighth House
It is time to withdraw and reassess where deep feelings or commitments are taking you.

Smoky quartz in northeast/Ninth House
More is happening than is apparent on the outside.

Smoky quartz in south/Tenth House
It is time to examine your dreams closely. How can you make them a reality?

Smoky quartz in northwest/Eleventh House
Now might be the time to avoid crowds and parties. You need some quiet time.

Smoky quartz in Twelfth House
Make sure that you have not overlooked any possibilities suggested by your dreams.

Personality
Smoky quartz people have a strong, quiet energy, and a deep, creative energy as well. Such a person may choose to lead a quiet life.

Energy
Potential, beginnings, change.

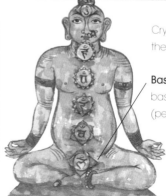

Crystals are placed on the base chakra.

Base (root) chakra
base of spine
(perineum)

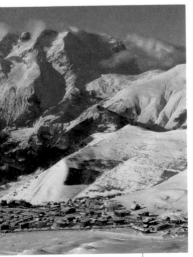

Above Like many minerals, smoky quartz is found in mountainous areas of the world. Erosion by wind, water, and frost gradually uncovers crystal-filled cavities in the rock.

Smoky quartz

Colour: yellow-brown to black

Hardness: 7

Composition: SiO_2 (silicon dioxide)

Qualities: quieting, grounding, protecting

Main chakra: base

Scotland, and is called "cairngorm" after the name of the mountain range in which it is found. Traditionally, fine examples of smoky quartz were polished and set as jewellery, and were handed down from generation to generation within a family as a protective or healing amulet.

Spiritual and healing properties

Smoky quartz has a gentle focusing and grounding energy. Whereas clear quartz enlivens and radiates light energy, smoky quartz absorbs and stores all energy. This type of quartz is useful in any situation where there is confusion or overactivity. It energises the grounding functions of the base chakra, so that the individual can focus on what is important. Smoky quartz also has a calming effect on the thought processes, and is an excellent stone for meditation. It can help to disperse fear and other negative states of mind and, because it creates stability in all body systems, it can provide security and protection.

Divinatory interpretation

Smoky quartz represents a stage of development where there is stillness. This can be right at the start, or even before the process of coming into being occurs. This stone is like the rich soil in which many things are able to grow when the time is right. In this context, it counsels patience and a very cautious level of activity, so as not to disturb the seeds of potential from sprouting.

At many stages of growth and development there are periods of quiescence, when nothing appears to be happening. Times like this indicate that change is under way at deep levels – probably well out of sight of everyday scrutiny. It is time to focus inwardly on plans and dreams, but do not settle or become fixed on any one outcome. Quiet contemplation, meditation, and withdrawal from outer activity can hasten the process.

Peacock Ore

A familiar mineral, peacock ore is best known for its bright surface colours of yellow, mauve, blue, and red.

P eacock ore is the common name for two related minerals, bornite and chalcopyrite. Both minerals are sulphides of iron and copper, and both commonly occur in copper-ore-bearing rocks. Chalcopyrite is a bright, brassy yellow colour, while bornite's colouration is more reddish brown. After the surface of either mineral has been exposed to some degree of weathering, a tarnish forms. This tarnish is comprised of assorted copper oxides or hydroxides, which form a thin layer over the mineral. When light strikes the tarnished surface, the result is a refraction into iridescent rainbow colours, similar to the effect of oil on water.

Myth and history

There is no doubt that peacock ore, as a primary ore of copper, has been known of since ancient times. Today, chalcopyrite is a primary industrial source of copper due to the fact that it is found in large quantities around the world; notable sources include Chile, Peru, Bolivia, Mexico, and the USA.

Spiritual and healing properties

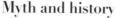

With its wide range of colours, peacock ore has the ability to stimulate each of the main chakras, as well as all of the subtle energy systems of the body. This process is helped along by the mineral's high copper content, which allows for a greater flow and integration of energy patterns.

Peacock ore

Colour: brassy yellow with bright blue, red, mauve
Hardness: 3–4
Composition: $CuFeS_4$ (chalcopyrite, sulfide of copper and iron)
Qualities: synthesizing, clearing
Main chakra: solar plexus

133

Suggested Crystal Readings

Peacock ore in centre/First House
An air of confidence will help to create an impression that others will trust.

Peacock ore in southeast/Second House
Find ways of being content with your financial and personal resources.

Peacock ore in east/Third House
When offering advice, make sure you are positive and supportive.

Peacock ore in north/Fourth House
Spend some time at home cleaning, tidying, and reorgansing in order to secure a base for yourself.

Peacock ore in west/Fifth House
Allow yourself to experience the joy of natural surroundings.

Peacock ore in Sixth House
Developing a positive outlook will help you to release the stress that has been building up.

Peacock ore in southwest/Seventh House
Start appreciating the value of your relationships and partnerships.

Peacock ore in Eighth House
Take time to pull together your diverse skills and focus them on a goal.

Peacock ore in northeast/Ninth House
Be open to whatever the universe offers you.

Peacock ore in south/Tenth House
Success is here, though you may not realise or appreciate it fully.

Peacock ore in northwest/Eleventh House
Spend time with those who share your views and philosophies on life.

Peacock ore in Twelfth House
Take time out to contemplate your potential and possibilities for growth.

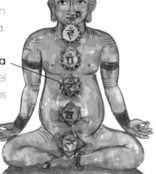

Crystals are placed on the solar plexus chakra.

Solar plexus chakra
midway between navel and base of ribs

Personality
Peacock ore is characterised by a mature and widely experienced person. This person is also enthusiastic, with an underlying confidence in life.

Energy
Joyful, integrated.

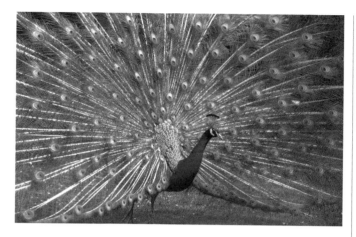

Left The name "peacock ore" is an old miner's term, yet it is undeniably an apt description of this stone, given that its intense iridescent colours do indeed resemble the plumage of a peacock.

Integration is one of the primary functions of this stone. The underlying golden colour relates directly to the solar plexus chakra, and thus peacock ore naturally encourages happiness and self-empowerment. It also provides protection from negativity. The presence of iron, copper, and sulphur hints at a strengthening of the circulatory and nervous systems, along with the physical structures of the body.

Below As a tool for healing, peacock ore can be used to lower calcium levels in the body, which can be helpful in treating arthritic conditions.

Divinatory interpretation

Peacock ore can improve the general outlook within any area in a reading because it has the power to bring all possibilities to bear. Just as peacock ore's wide variety of colours derives from the underlying gold-coloured rock, so a situation characterised by an underlying sense of contentment can lead to a variety of desirable outcomes.

Confidence is one of the main messages of this stone. Its appearance in a reading implies that success will be achieved in time, no matter what critics say. At this time, you should be able to integrate all aspects of the situation in a productive way.

Even in a difficult placement, peacock ore suggests that opportunities exist for happiness, as every experience, whether good or bad, creates new possibilities.

Bloodstone

Bloodstone is also known as heliotrope, and has a long tradition of magical use. A variety of chalcedony quartz, it has long been a valuable gemstone because of its striking red and green coloration.

Below Because of its dynamic energy, bloodstone is associated with the astrological sign Aries. Both are ruled by the planet Mars.

Bloodstone has the same chemical composition as green jasper, and is coloured by small crystals of actinolite and celedonite. The red spots, which resemble blood, are iron oxide. The most valuable bloodstone has distinct bright red patterns and comes from India, which has always been its primary source.

Myth and history

A thirteenth-century mystical text states that "A bat, represented on heliotrope or bloodstone, gives the wearer power over demons and helps incantations."

There were many ancient beliefs revolving around bloodstone, or heliotrope (meaning "turning toward the sun"), as it was called in ancient times. Various texts suggested that it could turn water red, darken the sun, or summon storms. It was also thought to have the power to stop the flow of blood from wounds and to confer strength, longevity, and honour to its wearer.

Bloodstone

Colour: green with red speckles
Hardness: 7
Composition: SiO_2 (quartz)
Qualities: circulating, supportive, motivating
Main chakra: heart, base

Spiritual and healing properties

The combined colours of bloodstone allow it to function at the levels of the base and heart chakras. It encourages a balance of energy; practicality, with the desire to

Suggested Crystal Readings

Bloodstone in centre/First House
You need to be seen to be making a practical effort within the situation.

Bloodstone in southeast/Second House
Consider carefully any personal expenditure, financial or energetic, before you act.

Bloodstone in east/Third House
Constructive ideas and suggestions can be very supportive.

Bloodstone in north/Fourth House
Your loyalty and support may be needed by family or close friends.

Bloodstone in west/Fifth House
New romance or projects that have been slow to start will blossom now.

Bloodstone in Sixth House
Courage is needed to break out into new areas and to start again.

Bloodstone in southwest/Seventh House
Rethink your motives if others get angry with you – are you manipulating them?

Bloodstone in Eighth House
Careful investment will pay off, but you need to be patient.

Bloodstone in northeast/Ninth House
Plans to broaden your experience can be made now, step by step.

Bloodstone in south/Tenth House
You need to appreciate the fact that success comes from planning and hard work.

Bloodstone in northwest/Eleventh House
Enthusiasm for group work will be strong but short-lived – unless you can gain from it.

Bloodstone in Twelfth House
Enforced periods of solitude or rest are likely needed to prevent exhaustion.

Personality
This stone represents a courageous, strong individual. This person is emotional, but is able to balance passion with calmness and understanding.

Energy
Courageous, strong, supportive.

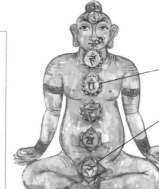

Crystals are placed on the heart and base chakras.

Heart chakra centre of breastbone in centre of chest and
Base (root) chakra Base of spine (perineum)

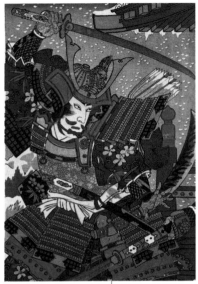

Above Warriors would often carry bloodstone into battle to prevent blood loss if injured.

Right Bloodstone has long been connected to the sun, as both are able to harness the power of life energy to create new possibilities in the world.

grow; calming, strong emotions; and is both stimulating and motivating. The heart and circulation is supported at a physical, energetic level. Spiritual qualities can be accessed and integrated into everyday life because the base chakra, the source of our life force, is activated in a controlled and disciplined way.

Divinatory interpretation

Bloodstone is connected to the sun and to the astrological sign Aries. This connection, along with its relation to the blood, links it to the qualities of strength, courage, and the energy to succeed against all odds.

In a reading, bloodstone suggests the need for perseverance and courage, but also implies that it is indeed possible to achieve your goals. In a difficult placement, bloodstone offers some protection from defeat. In a positive position, it can show that all obstacles will come to nothing, and that those around you will support you.

In situations of emotional turbulence, the presence of bloodstone may indicate the need to calm impulsive reactions, such as anger. Don't allow your heart to let you get carried away from reality.

Moldavite

Moldavite is a unique gemstone created by the explosive impact of meteorites millions of years ago.

Moldavite is the only gem-quality member of a small group of mysterious minerals known as tektites. Tektites are found throughout the world, and are thought to result from the massive heat and pressure waves generated by meteorite strikes on or close to the surface of the planet. They are glassy in composition, but have none of the trace elements expected from volcanic material. Most take the form of extruded drops, pebbles, and splatter shapes.

All tektites are opaque and earth-coloured with the exception of moldavites, which are found only in a small area of the Czech Republic, where they were formed some 15 million years ago. Deep, rich-green moldavites have been dug from sandpits, collected from fields, and used as ornaments and amulets for centuries. Most are small, with rippled and cratered surfaces.

Myth and history

This stone has been known to exist in central Europe for a long time, but it is only in the last couple of decades that any significant amounts have been made available. Unlike that of other gemstones, the volume of moldavite is finite – no other sources have been discovered and, as the product of some distant and unique event, another source is unlikely.

Moldavite is sometimes called an extraterrestrial stone, or a green meteorite. Tests show this to be unlikely, but there is no real consensus as to how tektite actually came into being.

Moldavite

Colour: glassy, bright green
Hardness: 5
Composition: amorphous silicates (glass)
Qualities: perceptive, intuitive
Main chakra: heart, throat, brow, crown

139

Suggested Crystal Readings

Moldavite in centre/First House
Others are likely to misunderstand or misread your intentions.

Moldavite in southeast/Second House
Sudden changes in personal finances or situations are possible at this time.

Moldavite in east/Third House
You need to speak up, even if it seems out of place and is out of character.

Moldavite in north/Fourth House
Upsets in the home are likely, but they are for the best in the long run.

Moldavite in west/Fifth House
Allow your sense of wonder to re-awaken – spend some time in natural surroundings.

Moldavite in Sixth House
Unexpected shifts in the way you work may open up new possibilities.

Moldavite in southwest/Seventh House
All relationships have their ups and downs. Don't take these fluctuations personally.

Moldavite in Eighth House
Open your eyes to the wider events going on in the world and how these control our lives.

Moldavite in northeast/Ninth House
Be open to all possibilities and probabilities – the sky is the limit.

Moldavite in south/Tenth House
Be prepared to stand out from the crowd and be labelled as such – for better or worse.

Moldavite in northwest/Eleventh House
Look closely at information concerning ecology, nature, and the environment for inspiration or guidance.

Moldavite in Twelfth House
Take time out to connect or reconnect with the Earth. This will help you to put everything into perspective.

Crystals are placed on the crown, brow, throat, and heart chakras.

Throat chakra neck

Crown chakra top of the head

Brow chakra centre of forehead

Heart chakra centre of breastbone in centre of chest

Yet those who have tuned into the energy of moldavite have been known to experience a series of strange, unearthly sensations, including speed, great heat, and a sense of expanded awareness.

Left The mysterious nature of moldavite has linked it to several powerful mystical objects, including the Holy Grail.

Spiritual and healing properties

Moldavite amplifies the qualities of any other stones nearby, emphasising their spiritual aspects. On its own, it activates the spiritual qualities of the heart chakra, particularly the relationship of the self to the universe and the quest for personal fulfilment. At the throat, brow, and crown chakras, moldavite enhances subtle perception, intuition, and visualization, and provides a fuller appreciation of existence.

Personality

The moldavite personality is strong and unconventional, and may have atypical or unpopular views. Big ideas and the desire to push the limits of experience are also characteristic.

Energy

Universal, expansive aware, awakened.

Divinatory interpretation

Moldavite's power comes from the violent forces unleashed when outer and inner space meet. Similarly, sometimes a shock is needed to make us realize that we have been living in a self-constructed dream of reality rather than in reality itself. Moldavite may indicate an awakening experience of any kind – not just one that is explosive. In either case, however, the result will be the same: a sudden broadening of experience and perception that changes our relationship to everything that is familiar. This may be difficult to deal with, or it may result in a natural feeling of opening up to new worlds.

Below A variety of tektites collected from sites in Texas, Vietnam, and Australia.

The presence of moldavite in a reading can also indicate a sudden and unexpected turn of events that can be the beginning of a great opportunity – assuming change is allowed to happen.

Jade

Although it is one of the hardest known minerals, jade – known also as jadeite and nephrite – has long been sought out as a stone for carving.

The name jade actually refers to two distinct minerals: jadeite and nephrite. Jadeite is slightly harder and has a deep-green colouring from impurities of chromium, whereas nephrite is softer and less dense.

As high-quality jade is uncommon, imitations are frequent; bowenite, a similar mineral to serpentine, is often stained green to imitate the rich colour of Imperial jade, while African jade is actually opaque green garnet, from the Transvaal region.

Jadeite

Colour: green
Hardness: 7
Composition: $NaAlSi_2O_6$ (jadeite)
Qualities: integrating, instinctual, aware
Main chakra: heart

Myth and history

Jade has a long and distinguished history, beginning at the dawn of civilization. Jade axe-heads of both ceremonial and ritual function have been found in Stone Age tombs. Some have been deliberately cut up or divided, suggesting a ritual of passing on the power of the deceased. In South America, jade was placed under the tongues of the dead. This practice was common in China, too, to protect the spirit of the deceased. The widespread use of jade in America was noted by the Spanish invaders, who brought many pieces back to Europe. They named the stone piedra de hijada, meaning "stone of the flank," because the Native Americans used it to treat kidney disease.

In China, jade was afforded the highest medicinal value. It was used to prolong life and strengthen the heart, lungs, voice, bones, and blood.

Suggested Crystal Readings

Jade in centre/First House
You have a need to appear to feel at home in any situation.

Jade in southeast/Second House
Trust yourself and follow your own beliefs and values.

Jade in east/Third House
It is a good idea to clarify how you feel and where you stand.

Jade in north/Fourth House
Inspiration can be found by looking at your family history.

Jade in west/Fifth House
You need to follow your own instincts when it comes to fun and enjoyment.

Jade in Sixth House
Continue to do things the way they have always been done.

Jade in southwest/Seventh House
Don't let your need to please others stop you from addressing your own needs.

Jade in Eighth House
When advice is given by those in authority, weigh it against your own gut reactions.

Jade in northeast/Ninth House
Make sure you know all the background history that has created the current situation.

Jade in south/Tenth House
Appreciate that where you are now is the result of many factors, not just your own efforts.

Jade in northwest/Eleventh House
Those who share the same roots as you can help you feel a sense of belonging.

Jade in Twelfth House
Examine any traditions that you follow or have adopted and make sure they fulfil your needs.

Personality
Jade represents those who are rooted in the traditions of family. There is a stability in these people that comes from a sense of continuity.

Energy
Stable, belonging, ancestral.

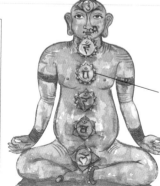

Crystals are placed on the heart chakra.

Heart chakra centre of breastbone in centre of chest

Nephrite

Colour: green, white, cream, brown

Hardness: 6–6.5

Composition: Ca(MgFe)$_5$Si$_8$O$_{22}$(OH)$_2$ (nephrite)

Qualities: integrating, instinctual, aware

Main chakra: heart

New Zealand is another important source of jade. The Maoris carved it into stylized human forms representing the ancestral spirits. Through these *hei-tiki*, meaning "carvings for the neck," the energy of the ancestors could be accessed by descendants' families.

Spiritual and healing properties

Jade has an overall balancing effect on the heart. It is a stabilising gemstone, as it helps bring awareness of the body's instinctual capacity. This level of awareness maintains a continual connection with the planet and its energies, creating a sense of belonging and an increased sensitivity to surroundings. Jade also improves the efficiency of all healing processes.

Right Jade not only has a long history. It has had uses in cultures across the world – from South America, to China and New Zealand.

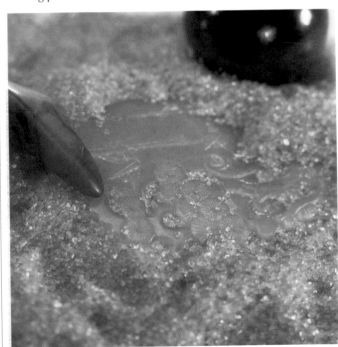

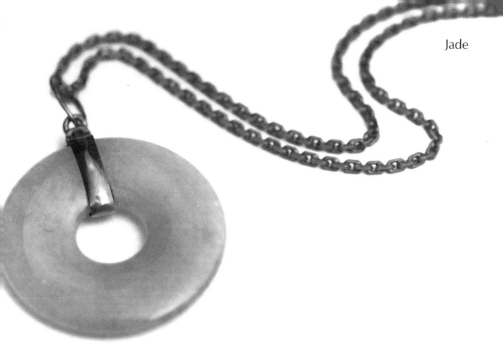

Divinatory interpretation

Jade provides an instinctive ability to sense the truth of any situation. In a reading, it may suggest that we should listen to our gut feelings more often. Jade's strength comes from its ability to connect the individual to the whole. It can therefore imply that we should either become more involved with a situation, or back off if our instincts tell us to do so.

As jade has a long relationship with the spirits of the dead, in a reading it can represent the traditions of our forebears. We are all connected to our ancestral genetic makeup, including its behavioural tendencies. Acknowledgment of this fact can provide insight into our personal lives.

Above Worn as jewellery, jade can improve the efficiency of all healing processes.

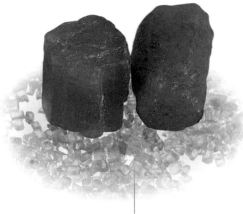

Emerald

Emerald is the quintessential green stone, yet it is rarely found free of faults or inclusions.

E merald is a rare variety of the mineral beryl, which forms in granite and pegmatite rocks, growing long, hexagonal prisms. Beryl crystals can grow extremely large – specimens that are several yards in length are not uncommon. The particular shade of green that makes beryl so sought after is caused by atoms of vanadium and chromium within the crystal lattice.

Emerald is a hard but brittle mineral, and commonly contains fractures, gas bubbles, droplets of water, and crystals of other minerals. In fact, emerald can be easily identified from these inclusions. Mica inclusions are common in African and Russian stones, and calcite and pyrite inclusions often appear in Brazilian stones.

The finest gem-quality emeralds come mainly from Colombia. The highest-quality stones required by the gem trade are very expensive, but nontransparent emerald crystals with visible inclusions and fractures can often be acquired at a reasonable cost. The difficulty of finding perfect emeralds has led gem-cutters to devise a special "emerald cut," where a rectangular stone is given long facets on the outside edges to emphasise the colour and disguise any imperfections.

Emerald

Colour: vivid green
Hardness: 7.5-8
Composition: $Be_3Al_2Si_6O_{18}$ (beryl, beryllium aluminium silicate)
Qualities: harmonious, cleansing, calming
Main chakra: heart

Right Faultless, clear emerald makes exceptional jewellery which encapsulates the green hues of the natural world.

Suggested Crystal Readings

Emerald in centre/First House
This stone shows the need to blend in and be at peace with your surroundings.

Emerald in southeast/Second House
Make sure that you truly appreciate and recognse what you have.

Emerald in east/Third House
Tell people you love how much you care, but don't expect them to reciprocate.

Emerald in north/Fourth House
"Home is where the heart is" – your sense of security stems from this adage.

Emerald in west/Fifth House
New romances and projects will benefit from your attention.

Emerald in Sixth House
You may need to consider changes at work if you don't really agree with what you are doing.

Emerald in southwest/Seventh House
Be loving with those in close relationships and open to everyone else.

Emerald in Eighth House
You have the skills to manage your own resources, if you trust yourself to do so.

Emerald in northeast/Ninth House
Share the wealth of your knowledge with those who care about the same issues.

Emerald in south/Tenth House
Pour your heart into the situation without expecting anything in return.

Emerald in northwest/Eleventh House
Friends are very important to you, as they can help you to keep your balance and perspective.

Emerald in Twelfth House
You need to be honest with yourself about your relationships regarding what you give and what you expect in return.

Personality

An emerald personality is open, clear-sighted, and loving. There is a quiet, strong energy, a conviction of the rightness of things, and an optimism borne of confidence and stability rather than wishful thinking.

Energy

Loving, optimistic, friendly.

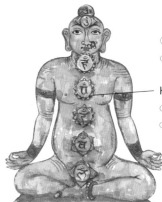

Crystals are placed on the heart chakra.

Heart chakra centre of breastbone in centre of chest

147

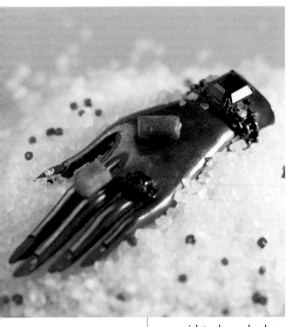

Myth and history

The ancient Egyptians mined emeralds south of Koseir, in Egypt. The green colour was associated with the life-giving properties of the River Nile and its surrounding vegetation. It became common practice to place an emerald in the mouth of a deceased person as they were mummified, so that they would spring up again in the afterlife. Green was the colour sacred to Osiris (Asar), the guide and guardian of human beings, and the god of fertility, agriculture, and abundance. Thoth (Tahuti), the god of knowledge, is said to have imparted his wisdom upon an emerald tablet.

In South America, the Peruvians are said to have had an emerald the size of an ostrich's egg, which they kept in a special temple to the goddess of the stone, making offerings of smaller emeralds. Many large, fine emeralds were brought to Europe by the Spanish after they conquered the Aztecs.

Throughout history, emerald has been connected with honesty, truth, and holiness. These qualities made it the primary stone to consider when proving the strength and genuineness of a relationship. Thus, emerald became a stone representing true love. It has also been used to refresh or improve eyesight, protect from snakebites and evil spirits, and bring on the skills of prophecy and foresight. The stone was said to shatter in the vicinity of wickedness and deceit.

Spiritual and healing properties

Emerald brings soothing harmony to all systems of the body, and speeds all cleansing and purifying processes. It can release hidden fears and anxiety, allowing the individual to experience finer spiritual states of awareness. Emerald can thus be a useful meditation stone. The rich green colour of the stone brings forth the energy of growth, peace, and abundance. The heart is the main area of balance for this stone.

Below Emerald was a symbol of life and knowledge to the ancient Egyptians.

Divinatory interpretation

Emerald in a reading indicates love, attachment, and true friendship. It requires an honest and open approach. Like emerald itself, even the finest relationship has fractures and imperfections. A true partnership is stronger than these faults, but a superficial relationship will shatter when placed under pressure.

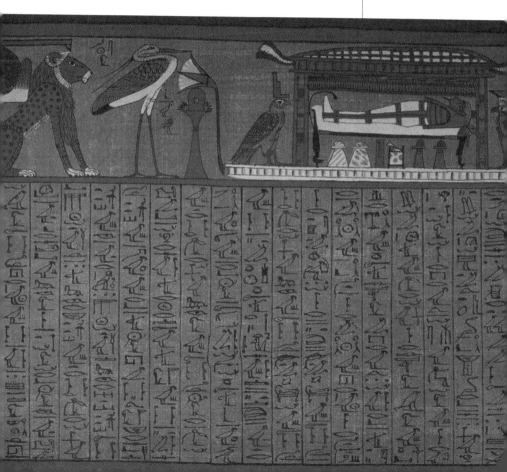

Aventurine

It is thought that this type of quartz, with its many colours and sparkling inclusions, derives its name from the Italian phrase *per avventura*, meaning "chance."

Aventurine forms when quartz melts and recrystallises in the presence of other minerals that colour the body of the rock. It is microcrystalline, and forms large slabs making it useful for creating ornamental objects.

Green aventurine is coloured by fuschite mica, which gives the stone a sprinkling of bright speckles. Although often subtle, this feature distinguishes it from similar-looking stones such as amazonite, emerald, and jade. Brown varieties take their colour from pyrites or goethite.

Aventurine

Colour: green, orange-brown
Hardness: 7
Composition: SiO_2 with inclusions
Qualities: tranquil, positive
Main chakra: solar plexus, heart

Myth and history

Aventurine has been valued by many civilizations over the centuries. Aventurine carvings from China date from the third century BC, and the stone was also used for carving in the Mediterranean area. Today aventurine remains a popular carving stone, particularly in India, China, and Brazil.

The origin of the present name for the stone may come from the Italian phrase *per avventura*, meaning "by chance" (thus implying that the discovery of the stone was accidental). It is also possible that the stone is named after a spangled type of decorative glass called *avventura*, which the stone resembles.

Right The calming qualities of aventurine make it particularly suitable for both meditation and emotional healing.

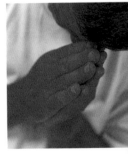

Suggested Crystal Readings

Aventurine in centre/First House
Enthusiasm to explore the situation could get excessive and end up scattering your focus.

Aventurine in southeast/Second House
Prudence and care with money will help you to resist the temptation to overspend.

Aventurine in east/Third House
Freedom of speech is crucial if you are to maintain your right to choose for yourself.

Aventurine in north/Fourth House
By making adjustments at home, you will gain more space or freedom.

Aventurine in west/Fifth House
Don't overlook the small possibilities in the bigger picture.

Aventurine in Sixth House
If you feel trapped, make minor changes to relieve the strain until you can really act.

Aventurine in southwest/Seventh House
New people in your life need time to get to know you – and time is needed for you to trust them.

Aventurine in Eighth House
Examine everything closely so you are clear about where you stand.

Aventurine in northeast/Ninth House
Taking a risk is probably worthwhile, but be on the lookout for unseen factors.

Aventurine in south/Tenth House
New avenues or directions may surface. Be cautious before committing yourself.

Aventurine in northwest/Eleventh House
You may feel like leaving the crowd behind to do things by yourself.

Aventurine in Twelfth House
Changing the way you think can be the easiest way to go about creating new situations out in the world.

Personality
The personality represented by this stone is optimistic, bright, and emotionally balanced, with clear insight. Perhaps this person is a practitioner of meditation that uses visual imagery.

Energy
Opportunity, chance, freedom.

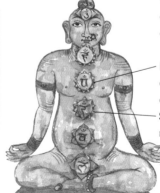

Crystals are placed on the solar plexus and heart chakras.

Heart chakra centre of breastbone in centre of chest

Solar plexus chakra midway between navel and base of ribs

151

Spiritual and healing properties

Green aventurine is perhaps the best balancing stone for the heart chakra. It encourages calmness and positivity, and helps to release emotional pain in a gentle, effective way. In any colour, aventurine is both a cleanser of negativity and an activator of positive life-supporting qualities. It can help to release childhood anxieties and fears, and is useful in certain spiritual practices, including meditation and creative visualization. In traditional Tibetan healing practices, aventurine is used for improving eyesight as well as clarity of insight, perception, and creativity.

The golden-brown varieties of aventurine work best at the level of the solar plexus, bringing increased self-confidence and an optimistic outlook on life.

Divinatory interpretation

When aventurine appears in a reading, it indicates that new opportunities may arise. Like the shining sparkles in the stone itself, these will need to be looked for carefully, and are most likely to appear where you least expect them to be.

In a positive placement, aventurine offers the chance of freedom, a sudden new departure, or a new road along which to travel. In a difficult placement, aventurine may suggest that the questioner is oblivious to certain opportunities to improve the current situation that are presenting themselves. More attention must be paid to details, as these may lead to a breakthrough.

Below Aventurine can help provide clarity of direction, thus presenting the opportunity to discover new life paths.

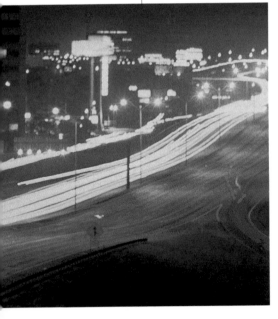

Malachite

Malachite is a copper ore. It has also been called "rock green," "the velvet ore," and "the satin ore," because of its striking colours and patterns.

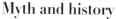

Malachite is a soft mineral often found in combination with blue zodiac. Both minerals are formed from the decomposition of copper ores exposed to water and air, making them good indicators of the presence of copper. Malachite rarely forms crystals, forming nodules instead that are a deep, silky green. Its concentric bands of colour make it a valuable decorative stone, despite its softness.

Myth and history

The name malachite derives from the Greek word for the mallow plant, *maloche*, the leaves of which are a similar shade of green.

Since classical times, malachite has been used as a protective amulet. Malachite carved with a sun's face was thought to provide protection from harm, evil spirits, and venomous animals. The concentric patterns of malachite often resemble an eye, and so, naturally, it was also used as a protection from the evil eye – the curse of a witch or an enemy. The ancient Egyptians mined the stone to use for decorative purposes and as a green pigment.

Malachite

Colour: concentric bands of light and dark green
Hardness: 3.5–4
Composition: $Cu_2CO_3(OH)_2$ (carbonate of copper)
Qualities: detoxifying, soothing
Main chakra: heart

Spiritual and healing properties

An absorbing stone, malachite is excellent for drawing out imbalances from the body. It has also been used to reduce the pain of inflammation, and can soothe minor aches and pains.

153

Suggested Crystal Readings

Malachite in centre/First House
Any jealousy or envy will be difficult to hide from others at the moment.

Malachite in southeast/Second House
Change your views as to why you think things are happening as they are.

Malachite in east/Third House
Take care that your immediate responses do not stem more from fear and anger than from logic.

Malachite in north/Fourth House
Older people's views may be at odds with your own. Allow them their opinions.

Malachite in west/Fifth House
Look for activities that you enjoy to reduce your stress levels.

Malachite in Sixth House
Don't ignore any health problems, particularly if they are inherited.

Malachite in southwest/Seventh House
Allow partners to soothe your fears.

Malachite in Eighth House
Forgive the people who seem to be responsible and your pain will ease.

Malachite in northeast/Ninth House
Spread your wings and break away from the thought patterns that have trapped you for so long.

Malachite in south/Tenth House
If you feel thwarted in your ambitions, look to your own assumptions for the cause.

Malachite in northwest/Eleventh House
You may need to develop your defences, as other people see you as the reason for their own upsets.

Malachite in Twelfth House
This is not a good time to manipulate situations behind the scenes, as you are seeing only part of the picture.

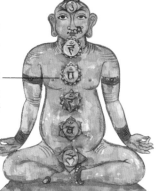

Crystals are placed on the heart chakra.

Heart chakra centre of breastbone in centre of chest

Personality

A positive malachite person is a healing, soothing character who will always help to ease another's pain, and will offer support in times of emotional turmoil. A negative malachite person is resentful, controlling, and difficult to trust.

Energy

Soothing, pain-relieving, calming.

Malachite is particularly effective at clearing emotional imbalances, and can bring peace and balance to the heart chakra. It also helps cleanse the body of toxins and pollutants. Care should be taken with malachite, however, as its dust is toxic if ingested.

Divinatory interpretation

In a reading, malachite suggests that there are many emotional levels which need to be taken into consideration, and signals that perhaps more care should be taken when dealing with emotional issues. As well, this stone intimates that letting go of old patterns, memories, and attachments is now necessary. Growth and the ability to move forward are contingent upon the ability to forgive – if not to forget. Painful situations must be understood, forgiven, and sent on their way. To do otherwise is to become trapped in the past.

In many ancient cultures, the evil eye was a common form of curse brought about by malevolent thoughts toward a person through jealousy or some other negative emotion. Make sure that you are not guilty of wishing harm upon others, and take care that you are not suffering yourself from strong negative emotions directed at you from nearby. Harbouring grudges and apportioning blame are life-damaging both to ourselves and to the person to whom the grudge and blame are directed.

Malachite teaches that there are many shades and levels to our actions. In a positive placement, it indicates a protected space, free from harm, in which it is possible to feel free and to grow.

Left Universally, the evil eye describes a look inspired by jealousy or maliciousness. In the past, especially when used by a witch or an enemy, it was thought to have the power to cause ills of all sorts, including bad luck and disease – even death.

Left The mallow plant, for which malachite is named, has the same properties as the stone: soothing and calming.

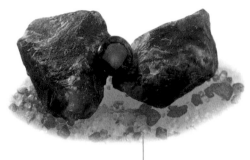

Moss Agate

Of all the wonderful variety within agate, moss agate is the most fascinating for its resemblance to the forms of living plants.

Moss agate

Colour: clear quartz with green and brown inclusions
Hardness: 6.5
Composition: SiO_2
Qualities: open, cleansing, optimistic
Main chakra: heart

Moss agate is transparent or translucent chalcedony quartz that has intergrown with crystals of manganese oxides, hornblende, and sometimes oxides of iron. These inclusions are usually green and brown, and take a dendritic form – that is, they resemble plant forms in the way they grow.

Myth and history

Moss agate was once known as "mocha stone," after one of the main sources of the mineral, the town of Al Mukna (Mocha) on the Red Sea coast of Yemen. It has long been sought for ornamental uses such as cameo brooches, rings, and vases.

Right A wonderful vehicle for attuning to the Earth, moss agate is a particularly useful stone for gardeners.

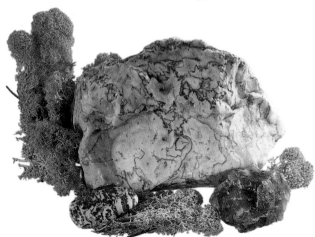

Suggested Crystal Readings

Moss agate in centre/First House
You need to make a new start, to find space, and to be yourself.

Moss agate in southeast/Second House
Look for new ways to get what you have always wanted.

Moss agate in east/Third House
It is time to listen to what people are really saying rather than what you think they are saying.

Moss agate in north/Fourth House
Personal space is paramount now. Certain steps are required to insure you get it.

Moss agate in west/Fifth House
Time spent outdoors will help rekindle your enjoyment of life.

Moss agate in Sixth House
You need to make changes to your work environment so that you feel more comfortable.

Moss agate in southwest/Seventh House
Say what is in your heart. Share your feelings.

Moss agate in Eighth House
Restrictions imposed by society may be obstructing your choices.

Moss agate in northeast/Ninth House
Choices on offer are not binding forever. Opportunities will come again.

Moss agate in south/Tenth House
Look for ways to broaden your approach to your work and ambitions.

Moss agate in northwest/Eleventh House
Reach out to new friends and develop new areas of interest.

Moss agate in Twelfth House
Make time to be alone and reflect on your life. Choices and directions will be clarified this way.

Crystals are placed on the heart chakra.

Heart chakra centre of breastbone in centre of chest

157

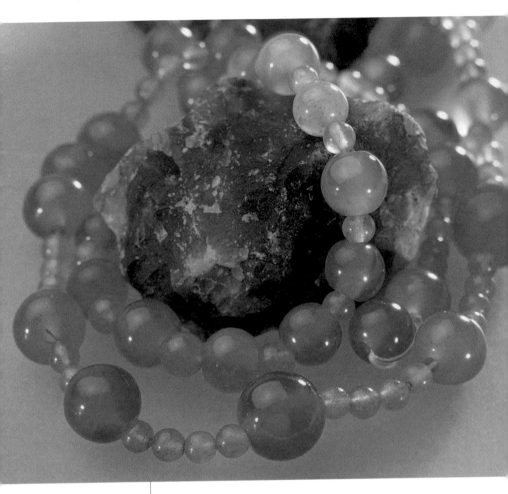

Spiritual and healing properties

The green colouring within moss agate naturally aligns its energy with the heart chakra. The treelike patterns are also reminiscent of the fine airways of the lungs and the small capillary blood vessels, as well as the channels of the lymphatic system. Where there is congestion and constriction in the lungs, blood, or lymph supplies, moss agate will help to free up those passageways. It can also be useful for detoxification processes.

158

Moss agate encourages openness within the mind and emotions, creating feelings of expansion, freedom, and space. These feelings create confidence and the desire to experience new things in life.

Due to its natural-looking shapes and predominant colours, moss agate resonates with all realms of nature. It also encourages awareness of the natural world and helps plant growth.

Divinatory interpretation

Moss agate brings the spirit of the natural world into a reading, and may suggest that spending more time enjoying the open spaces and green silence of the countryside would be beneficial. Because an escape to the countryside is a well-known antidote to overwork, tension, and other constricting circumstances of an urban lifestyle, the appearance of this stone may imply that stress is a current problem in the questioner's life. This stress may stem from a sense of duty or obligation; a difficult and demanding job; emotional or relationship problems causing insecurity or indecision; or feelings of being trapped. In order to come to terms with these restrictions, space and balance of mind are required.

In our lives, we are usually offered a choice of paths down which to travel; this stone suggests that the time has come to choose a path and move along it. Even a short distance away, a problem can cease to look like an insurmountable obstacle. Whatever the problem, moss agate implies that it's time to gain some perspective.

Personality

The moss agate person is a free spirit. He or she is at ease with nature, and is able to make do with whatever resources are available. This individual is a poet or dreamer, and can't stand to be pinned down or restricted by outside constraints.

Energy

Natural, curious, spacious.

Left The many treelike, branching structures within the human body all respond well to the presence of moss agate, which helps to relieve constriction and blockages.

159

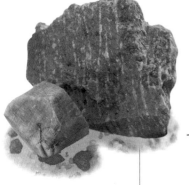

Amazonite

Amazonite is a variety of feldspar, the most common mineral within the Earth's crust.

Feldspar is a complex family of related minerals that includes many colourful and useful stones. Amazonite is one of the most easily identified members of the feldspar family because of its characteristic blue-green colour. The mineral name for amazonite is microcline. Amazonite crystals are easy to identify, forming flat, columnar prisms that are clearly bounded, substantial-looking, and often intergrown.

Amazonite derives its name from the Amazon River in South America, even though it is jade, not amazonite, that is found there. A popular semiprecious gemstone, amazonite is commonly used for cabochons and beads. It is easily identified by its mottled, streaky, or parallel lines of lighter and darker greens, caused by atoms of lead within the crystal lattice.

Amazonite

Colour: blue-green, with lighter striations
Hardness: 6–6.5
Composition: $KAlSi_3O_8$ (potassium aluminosilicate)
Qualities: calming, communicative
Main chakra: throat, heart

Myth and history

The ancient Egyptians often used amazonite, or *uat*, as they called it, for carvings. Its colour resembles turquoise – sometimes even emerald and jade. The colours of these stones were commonly associated with the afterlife, fertility, and protection from harm.

Amazonite is thought to have been among the stones in the Hebrew high priest's breastplate, as described in the book of Exodus.

Spiritual and healing properties

The colour of amazonite aligns it to the heart and throat chakras. It is a calming stone that helps to balance and stabilize the

Suggested Crystal Readings

Amazonite in centre/First House
You need to appear open-minded and interested in all possibilities.

Amazonite in southeast/Second House
Financial factors are crucial to your current situation.

Amazonite in east/Third House
Communicate clearly and precisely what you feel and think.

Amazonite in north/Fourth House
The foundations need to be further strengthened in order to support any more expansion.

Amazonite in west/Fifth House
Try new hobbies or learn new skills in order to broaden your knowledge base and to provide yourself with greater options.

Amazonite in Sixth House
Keep an outward, big-picture outlook on work, even if the going is tough.

Amazonite in southwest/Seventh House
Use a buoyant and optimistic approach in any sort of relationship discussion, but always be truthful.

Amazonite in Eighth House
Obstacles will be highlighted so that you can deal with them easily.

Amazonite in northeast/Ninth House
Keep your options open until you find something that really suits you.

Amazonite in south/Tenth House
Be prepared to step away from your usual routine and toward new experiences.

Amazonite in northwest/Eleventh House
Your opinion is needed in social situations.

Amazonite in Twelfth House
Restlessness may be intense, and you may feel trapped. If you relax, it will pass quickly.

Personality

An amazonite is an inquisitive person, always investigating the unknown and interested in a wide range of subjects. The amazonite person is also a good communicator and an intellectual.

Energy

Outgoing, curious.

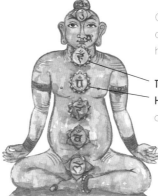

Crystals are placed on the throat and heart chakras.

Throat chakra neck
Heart chakra centre of breastbone in centre of chest

161

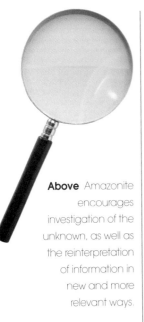

nervous system. Communication, memory, and brain functions are all enhanced by amazonite.

Like many turquoise and green stones, amazonite has been used to stimulate psychic skills and subtle sensitivity. It is sometimes even able to rekindle awareness of events from the distant past, known as "far memory." The images and sensations arising from far memory often relate in some way to the current life circumstances of the individual experiencing them.

Divinatory interpretation

Above Amazonite encourages investigation of the unknown, as well as the reinterpretation of information in new and more relevant ways.

The energies of the heart and throat combine in this stone to positively affect personal expression and creativity. In a reading, amazonite is related to sharing points of view, standing up and being counted, and the exploration of new experiences.

Amazonite indicates an outgoing, expansive phase of life motivated by a sincere desire to understand and to learn. It also seeks to clarify where the individual is in his or her life, and what his or her purpose is in the world. This stone suggests that this is the time to embark on projects or challenges long dreamed about but never tried, to expand our horizons, and to dare to be a little different.

Right Precious metals and gemstones can often be found deposited along the length of great rivers such as the Amazon. These materials require no elaborate mining to recover – just patience and a good eye.

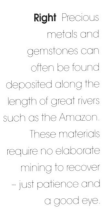

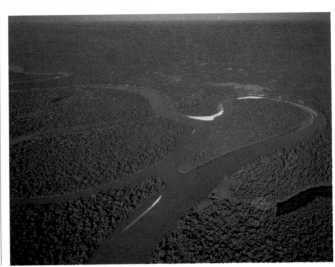

Aquamarine

Aquamarine is the precious, clear blue-green variety of the mineral beryl.

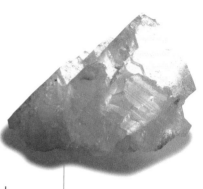

L ike all beryls, aquamarine is found in pegmatites, and can grow into large, hexagonal crystals. Often, these crystals contain thin, parallel cavities of gas and water and, as with other beryls, inclusions of mica and iron oxides are common.

Aquamarine shows dichroism; that is, the rich blue colour seen from some angles almost disappears when seen from others. This characteristic can help to identify the many imitations of this crystal. Iron atoms within the lattice are the source of aquamarine's blue colour. Because most jewellers prefer very particular shades of blue crystals, the less popular shades can be inexpensive to acquire.

Aquamarine

Colour: blue, blue-green
Hardness: 7.5–8
Composition: $Be_3Al_2Si_6O_{18}$ (beryl)
Qualities: expressive, cleansing
Main chakra: throat

Myth and history

The colour of aquamarine has connected it to the element of water, and to the sea in particular. From the third century BC, Greeks and Romans used the stone as a protective charm for overseas journeys, together with cameos carved with images of Poseidon, god of the sea, with his trident. Aquamarine was also a symbol of happiness and hope and, like emerald, was associated with love and friendship.

Left The colours within aquamarine so closely resemble the colours of the sea that in ancient times the stone quickly became associated with the deities of the sea.

163

Suggested Crystal Readings

Aquamarine in centre/First House
Be willing to offer companionship and support.

Aquamarine in southeast/Second House
Examine your own motivations before you blame others.

Aquamarine in east/Third House
Circumstances may require that you spend a lot of time talking.

Aquamarine in north/Fourth House
Do not ignore those at home in favour of a busy social life.

Aquamarine in west/Fifth House
Get out there and have some fun with friends.

Aquamarine in Sixth House
Do not take your work too seriously. Help others to keep the atmosphere light.

Aquamarine in southwest/Seventh House
There may be celebrations with close friends in your near future.

Aquamarine in Eighth House
Others really need you to be around to support them at this time.

Aquamarine in northeast/Ninth House
Travel over water for leisure purposes may be in your future.

Aquamarine in south/Tenth House
Insure that your plans include everyone who wants to join you.

Aquamarine in northwest/Eleventh House
Gossip may be clouding relationships with friends or other groups of people.

Aquamarine in Twelfth House
Take a few steps back so that you can see what is really going on.

Crystals are placed on the throat chakra.

Throat chakra
neck

Personality

Aquamarine represents a friendly, supportive, talkative person who is full of stories and ideas. This person might be connected to the sea or to seafaring in some way.

Energy

Companionable, convivial.

Spiritual and healing properties

Aquamarine can provide a significant boost to the immune system. It has a cleansing action that, in combination with its ability to stimulate the thymus gland, can help clear infection from the body. It may, however, bring old symptoms to the surface before they are finally released.

The throat chakra is energized by this crystal, encouraging creative expression and communication skills. There is also an improvement in mood, with an increase in hopefulness, optimism, and inspiration.

Divinatory interpretation

Aquamarine is a sign of communication in a reading. The interpretation of the reading will depend on whether the stone is located in a favourable or a difficult position. In a favourable position, this stone suggests companionship, conviviality, and a sharing of joy and optimism with loved ones. When surrounded by difficult energies, however, aquamarine may suggest that thoughtless gossip or the spreading of lies is causing problems. It may also indicate deception. Like imitations of the stone itself, this sort of behaviour will become clear if you patiently examine the situation from many different angles. It is important, though, not to become too emotionally involved – in other words, keep your cool. In some positions, aquamarine may also suggest travel over water.

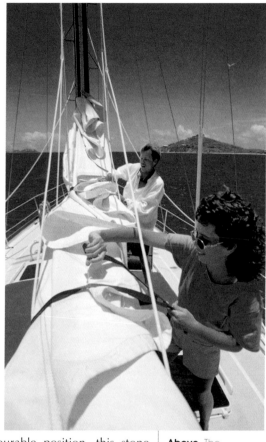

Above The invigourating effects of the sea have been noted for centuries. Similarly stimulating effects are attributed to the aquamarine crystal.

165

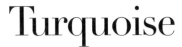

Turquoise

In many ancient cultures, turquoise was used as an amulet for protection and was a symbol of wealth.

T urquoise is created when water comes into contact with, and acts upon, a combination of copper and aluminium minerals. The resulting crystals are very small, and usually occur in massive form or granules. The stone's blue colour derives from its copper content, whereas the green tones are due to impurities. It is easy to identify turquoise from different areas by appearance – even individual mines can often be recognised from the appearance of the stones.

Turquoise is very porous, and easily absorbs dirt and oils. Heat and sunlight will often change its colour. To stabilise its colour and reduce its porousness, turquoise is often impregnated with a wax or resin.

Turquoise
Colour: light blue, blue-green, green
Hardness: 5-6
Composition: $CuAl_6(PO_4)_4(OH)_8$ 4-5H_2O (hydrated phosphate of aluminium and copper)
Qualities: strengthening, supportive
Main chakra: throat

Myth and history

Turquoise was mined by the ancient Egyptians in the Sinai Peninsula, near the Red Sea. It was also mined in Persia. The Ottoman Turks valued the stone and, despite some turquoise being found in Anatolia, they continued the often difficult trading process with the tribes controlling the mining operations. This demand for turquoise made it an expensive and valuable commodity. It entered the European markets via Turkey, and thus, from the thirteenth century onward, it became known as "turquoise," the Turkish stone.

Suggested Crystal Readings

Turquoise in centre/First House
Be wary and cautious in the ways in which you respond to people and events.

Turquoise in southeast/Second House
Your energy levels may not be at their best, so learn to pace yourself.

Turquoise in east/Third House
Say what you mean to say, not what someone else wants to hear.

Turquoise in north/Fourth House
Double-check your security at home. Emotional boundaries may need some attention.

Turquoise in west/Fifth House
Allow your instincts to guide your creative activities.

Turquoise in Sixth House
Pay attention to your health. Eat well, and don't overwork yourself.

Turquoise in southwest/Seventh House
Do not ignore your own wishes when making decisions.

Turquoise in Eighth House
Be careful not to exceed your budget at the moment.

Turquoise in northeast/Ninth House
Teachers and guides can help you clarify your thoughts and feelings.

Turquoise in south/Tenth House
Make sure you have a secure fallback position.

Turquoise in northwest/Eleventh House
Friends can help you to regain your sense of security.

Turquoise in Twelfth House
Take time to explore the spiritual aspects of your life.

Personality
Self-contained and assured, the turquoise personality is skilled in the physical world, but also has a firm foundation in the spirit world. He or she is likely a teacher, healer, or guide.

Energy
Immune, protective.

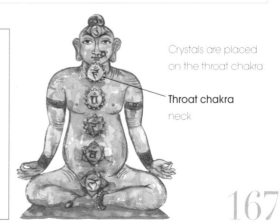

Crystals are placed on the throat chakra.

Throat chakra
neck

167

In Persia, turquoise was used to protect men and horses from falls and injuries. A thirteenth-century Persian book on the virtues of stones says, "Whoever owns the true turquoise set in gold will not injure any of his limbs when he falls, whether he be riding or walking, so long as he has the stone with him."

Historically, turquoise was a popular stone in Europe, and was typically worn by men as a gemstone set in rings. The Native American peoples – particularly in the southwestern states, where turquoise is found – valued the stone as a hunting aid. They also used it as a tool for healers and shamans, and for protection against harm. The Aztecs and Mayas used turquoise as an offering to the gods, and in China and Tibet, turquoise has long been worn as a protective amulet, and in a jewellery format as a sign of wealth.

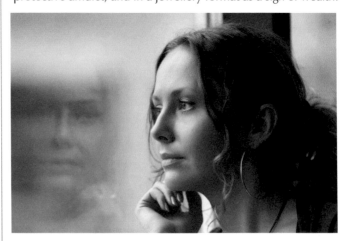

Spiritual and healing properties

As a blue stone with a hint of green, turquoise works naturally at the level of the heart and throat chakras. In particular, it stimulates the subtle energies of the thymus gland, midway between the heart and throat, an area which plays an important part in the body's immune system. Turquoise also acts as a general strengthener for all systems of the body, and offers protection from harm by ensuring a high level of energy function. The effects of environmental pollution and negativity are reduced and, as with many green- and turquoise-coloured stones, psychic sensitivity and connection with the spirit world are enhanced.

Divinatory interpretation

Turquoise appearing in a reading suggests the need to take precautions for personal safety. Be wary, be alert, and be prepared to deal with whatever unforeseen difficulties may arise. This is not an indication of danger; it is simply a warning that the situation requires care and extra attention.

In a positive placement, turquoise can show that everything is working in harmony; all factors are balanced, and there is a general optimistic atmosphere. Turquoise also suggests that, in order for things to work at optimum levels, you must communicate your feelings and preferences. Where health is an issue, turquoise may indicate a need to monitor the level of present environmental stresses, including pollution, electromagnetic radiation, noise, as well as negative emotions.

Below In this Tibetan brooch, the powers of the heavens, represented by turquoise, are united with those of the Earth, represented by rubies.

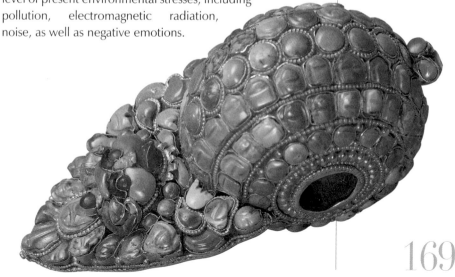

169

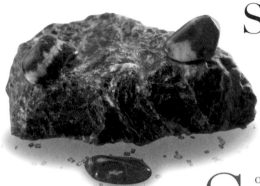

Sodalite

Sodalite can be easily confused with its relative, lapis lazuli. The two crystals are sometimes found together.

Sodalite derives its name from its high sodium content, and is related to several other aluminosilicates with very similar structures. It is commonly found in massive, microcrystalline form; crystals are rare. The deep-blue varieties have long been popular as gemstones, and are sometimes used as an alternative to lapis lazuli, although sodalite can be distinguished from lapis lazuli fairly easily by its white veining, its slightly darker blue colour, and its lack of pyrites.

Sodalite
Colour: deep blue with white veins and inclusions
Hardness: 5.5–6
Composition: $Na_4Al_3Si_3O_{12}Cl$ (aluminosilicate of sodium with chlorine)
Qualities: peaceful, clarifying, perceptive
Main chakra: throat, brow

Myth and history

Sodalite was not identified as a separate mineral until the nineteenth century. It has, however, been used for many centuries for making beads. No doubt it would have been named "sapphire" in the Middle Ages, as virtually all deep-blue gemstones were.

Spiritual and healing properties

Sodalite works well in unison with the throat and brow chakras. It is a clarifying stone that balances the emotions and steadies the thought processes. Like all deep-blue stones, it will bring a deep level of peace, and thus can be a useful aid to meditation and contemplation.

The white veining in sodalite is suggestive of communications with far-flung parts of the universe. Sodalite also helps to

Suggested Crystal Readings

Sodalite in centre/First House
You may find yourself in the role of mediator or peace-broker.

Sodalite in southeast/Second House
Learn to accept yourself as you are.

Sodalite in east/Third House
Be prepared to act as the go-between for various groups of people.

Sodalite in north/Fourth House
Do what you can to create peace at home.

Sodalite in west/Fifth House
You have plenty of time for relaxation and leisure. Enjoy yourself.

Sodalite in Sixth House
New opportunities at work need to be firmly grasped.

Sodalite in southwest/Seventh House
Listen to what others are saying before expressing your own opinions.

Sodalite in Eighth House
Others may be tempting you to take up new financial commitments. Think hard before you do anything and don't overextend yourself.

Sodalite in northeast/Ninth House
Make sure that your message is being heard by as many people as possible.

Sodalite in south/Tenth House
Be prepared to expand your horizons further than you had ever thought possible.

Sodalite in northwest/Eleventh House
You may be expected to resolve disputes by talking to everyone involved.

Sodalite in Twelfth House
Pay attention to your instincts, intuition, and dreams.

Personality
A typical sodalite individual has strong links to communication technologies. His or her primary interest likely lies in the exchange of information. This person is also emotionally restrained and self-possessed.

Energy
Mediator, communicator.

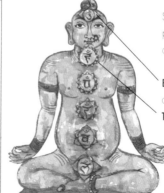

Sodalite crystals are placed on the brow and throat chakras.

Brow chakra at the centre of forehead
Throat chakra at the neck

support the lymphatic system, and thus the immune functions of the body. Its high sodium content benefits the body's fluid systems.

Divinatory interpretation

The appearance of sodalite in a reading indicates communication on a large scale – both between different peoples and between distant countries. Messages are constantly being sent and received using a variety of methods, including wires, cables, the airwaves, and satellites – even telepathically, between minds.

Sodalite also acts as a mediator and peace-bringer, and its appearance in a reading represents a meeting of minds. Expect news that will bring resolutions and new opportunities, but you must be ready to play your part. If you are not receiving the messages you expect, it may be necessary to contact others involved in the situation and to keep talking about the issue.

Sodalite in a reading can also suggest a state of peace and contentment, but not one of isolation. You may be by yourself, but you will not feel alone. This can be an ideal opportunity for research and study.

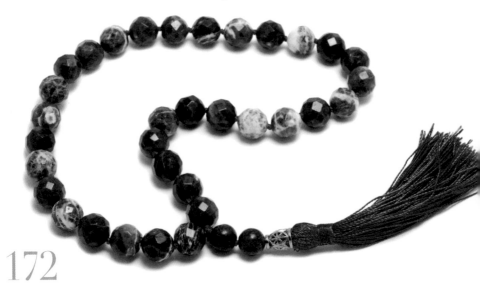

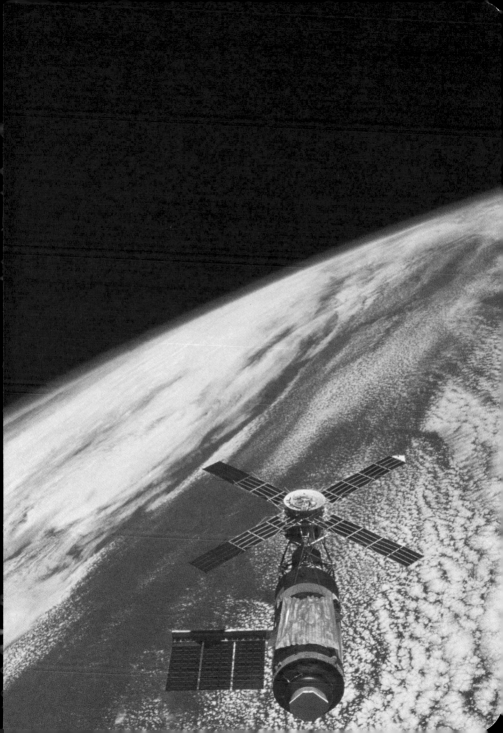

Lapis Lazuli

Lapis lazuli is a precious deep-blue rock containing lazurite, along with other minerals.

Lapis lazuli forms when limestone comes into contact with calcite and pyrite, creating a new, deep-blue mineral known as lazurite. A rock rather than a single mineral, lapis usually consists of compact lazurite crystals peppered with white dolomite, calcite, grains of pyrite, and sodalite. Lazurite crystals by themselves are less common than lapis lazuli rock.

Myth and history

The best source for lapis lazuli has always been Afghanistan, where the finest deep-blue stones are mined. Chile is a good source as well; other sites include Italy, Russia, and Argentina.

The name of this precious stone derives from the Latin for stone, lapis, and the Persian name of the mineral, *lajuward*, from which the word "azure" also derives. Some ancient authorities used the name sapphirus or "sapphire" when talking about lapis.

Called *chesbet* by the ancient Egyptians, lapis lazuli was sacred to Maat, the goddess of truth and balance, and was worn by the chief priest to invoke that goddess's power of justice. The Egyptians also used lapis lazuli

Right The ceremonial vestments of the Egyptian pharoahs were often adorned with lapis lazuli, which was seen as a symbol of divine justice.

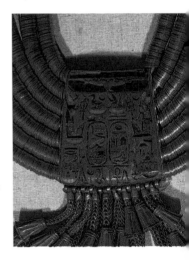

Suggested Crystal Readings

Lapis lazuli in centre/First House
It is important that you be impartial and fair in your dealings.

Lapis lazuli in southeast/Second House
Be cautious when judging people or situations by your own standards.

Lapis lazuli in east/Third House
Do not get drawn into gossiping about others.

Lapis lazuli in north/Fourth House
Distant memories may be very helpful in putting current events into perspective.

Lapis lazuli in west/Fifth House
Take time out to appreciate the beauty of natural surroundings.

Lapis lazuli in Sixth House
Don't rush into sudden decisions without first making sure you have all the facts.

Lapis lazuli in southwest/Seventh House
Honesty is needed from both partners in a current relationship.

Lapis lazuli in Eighth House
It will take some effort to uncover the truth of the situation.

Lapis lazuli in northeast/Ninth House
You need to stand up for the truth, even if this means you will be standing alone.

Lapis lazuli in south/Tenth House
Don't step on people to achieve your goals. The consequences will damage your ambitions.

Lapis lazuli in northwest/Eleventh House
Be careful to avoid excess of all kinds in your social life.

Lapis lazuli in Twelfth House
You need to find a peaceful space away from the busy world.

Personality

The lapis lazuli person is a serious, deep thinker, perhaps a teacher of some kind, but at an advanced level. He or she may also be involved with the law.

Energy

Truthful, serious.

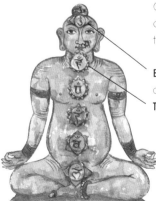

Crystals are placed on the brow and throat chakras.

Brow chakra centre of forehead
Throat chakra neck

175

to carve scarabs and cylinders, as well as for decorating royal vestments and temples. Roman soldiers wore lapis lazuli scarabs in rings for courage and protection. The stone was also ground up to make the pigment known as ultramarine.

Spiritual and healing properties

Lapis lazuli is a deep balancer, and works especially well with the brow and throat areas. It can remove deep levels of stress and trauma from the system, although some discomfort during the clearing process may be experienced.

Lapis brings the spiritual qualities of deep silence and perspective that can be unnerving to those unfamiliar with these sensations. It is in this space, however, that profound intuition and inspiration can arise.

Lapis lazuli can also help access levels of universal truth and balance that reach far beyond individual concepts of right and wrong, and is excellent for the healing of deep or chronic wounds of all sorts.

Divinatory interpretation

In a reading, lapis lazuli shows that truth is essential in the situation if success is to be achieved. Honesty, straightforward communication, and clarity will allow all energies to flow easily. It may also reveal the necessity to dig deep in order to uncover the truth of a situation. As a stone of the goddess of truth and balance, in some instances it may show the workings of law and order in society.

A stone of teaching, lapis lazuli may also indicate a time of study or of learning. In a position related to individual spirituality, it shows deep reflection, meditation, working with the distant past, and significant memories. Wherever it appears, lapis lazuli is a sobering, balancing, and profound influence.

Facing Page
Cosmic balance and personal virtue were united in Egyptian beliefs regarding the soul's journey in the afterlife. Lapis lazuli was thought to help the dead pass safely through their trials.

Lapis lazuli

Colour: deep blue with white and gold flecks
Hardness: 5.5
Composition: $(Na, Ca)_8$ $(Al, Si)_{12} O_{24} (S, SO_4)$ (sodium aluminosilicate with sulphur)
Qualities: consciousness, memory, meditation
Main chakra: throat, brow

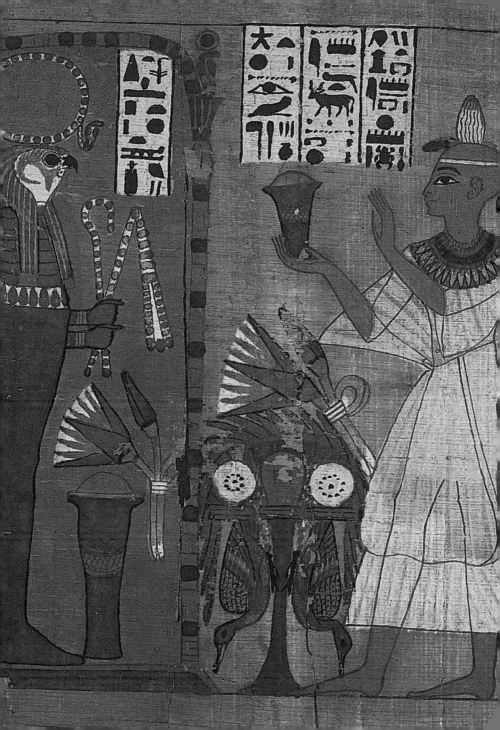

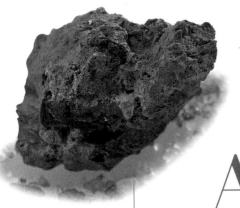

Azurite

Electric-blue azurite crystals have long been a valuable source of pigment for artists.

Azurite is a secondary mineral, forming from the oxidation of copper ores. Over time, as it absorbs water, it changes into the green mineral malachite. The two minerals are thus often found together in the ground, and can form an azurite-malachite rock that is blue-green in colour.

Crystals of azurite are rare but extremely beautiful, with deep blue blades catching the light on their edges, and showing a stunning, electric-blue colour. Most commonly, azurite appears as a powdery concretion in a lighter, forget-me-not shade of blue. Although an ore of copper, azurite is rarely used as a commercial source of that metal.

Myth and history

Azurite is named for its colour, "azure" blue. Ancient metalworkers and miners would have recognised this mineral, and would likely have known that workable copper could probably be found nearby.

Azurite has been used as an ornamental stone and a gemstone despite its softness, simply because of its wonderful colour. When found together with malachite, azurite tends to be a little more robust.

In the early Middle Ages and early Renaissance, azurite was used to make blue pigments called "mountain blue" and "Armenian stone." Over time, these pigments can collect water and change from blue to green, which is why many of the paintings from the thirteenth century have such an unusual colour scheme today.

Azurite

Colour: blue, dark blue
Hardness: 3.5–4
Composition: $Cu_3(CO_3)_2 (OH)_2$
Qualities: integration, consciousness, understanding
Main chakra: brow

Suggested Crystal Readings

Azurite in centre/First House
Try to be more open to the opinion of others.

Azurite in southeast/Second House
Allow change to happen, even though you are uncertain of the outcome.

Azurite in east/Third House
Keep things running smoothly with prompt communications.

Azurite in north/Fourth House
Try to relax, even though events may be moving faster than you feel comfortable with.

Azurite in west/Fifth House
Take time to explore activities that bring a sense of peace.

Azurite in Sixth House
The giving or receiving of a healing touch is required at the moment.

Azurite in southwest/Seventh House
This is a time to be close to those you care about. Listen to their concerns.

Azurite in Eighth House
Sensitivity to others' feelings will help you pinpoint areas that need healing.

Azurite in northeast/Ninth House
Make it your goal to learn more about healing techniques that interest you.

Azurite in south/Tenth House
You need to seriously consider a complete change of direction and a transformation of your goals.

Azurite in northwest/Eleventh House
Lingering unresolved issues need to be dealt with.

Azurite in Twelfth House
Experiment with techniques that calm the mind and relax the body.

Personality

The azurite person is a healer – perhaps by profession, or perhaps in everyday behaviour with others. This person can always lift a situation to the highest possible level, and is both mysterious and enigmatic.

Energy

Healing, transformative, empathetic.

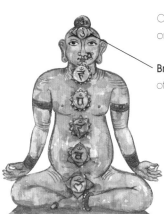

Crystals are placed on the brow chakra.

Brow chakra centre of forehead.

179

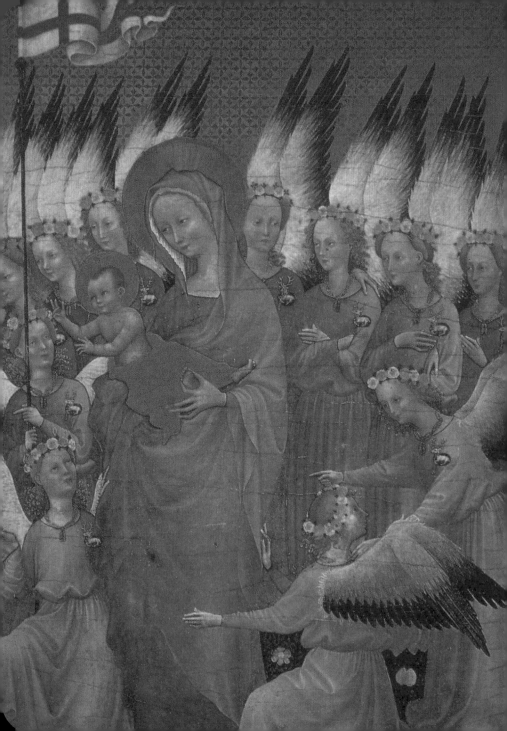

Spiritual and healing properties

The dark brilliance of azurite speeds the vibration of all energies toward the spiritual realm. Blue stones tend to be quietening and cooling, but azurite has a shifting, transformative quality. It is also known to stimulate deep levels of consciousness, and to increase subtle communication skills such as intuition, creativity, and inspiration. Understanding is also encouraged.

Azurite also has the ability to release deep stresses, and can help heal ailments caused by a breakdown of communication between different bodily systems. Security and an increased ease of energy flow make azurite an important stone for healers, as well as for those who wish to develop their own healing skills.

Divinatory interpretation

Azurite in a reading will bring swift results to the area in which it appears. It has the ability to smooth over and transform difficult and rigid circumstances, encouraging understanding and acceptance at deep healing levels.

In areas of conflict, azurite suggests that a resolution is within reach. It will bring a deepening level of awareness, establishing a quiet but dynamic stability and assuredness. In situations that have been locked or stuck, azurite suggests that changes are about to occur, and that a newer, more creative flow of energy is about to begin.

Azurite tells us as well that increased communication and understanding can bring forth a deep empathy which may help to resolve conflict. Transformation and change may also occur, so it is necessary to remain both flexible and aware.

Above Traditionally, the intense blue colour of azurite insured its use as a pigment for making paints.

Facing Page The Virgin Mary, dressed in blue robes, is an archetypal image of a healer. With its rich blue colouration, azurite is an important stone for healers.

Sapphire

Sapphire is the blue variety of the mineral corundum, one of the hardest of all stones.

Sapphire is the name given to all types of corundum except for the red variety, which is called ruby. Although the blue stone is the most well known and highly prized, sapphires also occur in yellow and white, although these colours often turn blue upon heating. The rich colouration of blue sapphire is caused by impurities of iron and titanium oxides within the crystal matrix.

This crystal is characteristically barrel-shaped, with six sides. It is found in metamorphic rocks that have been subjected to great heat and pressure, and also in alluvial deposits, where the bedrock has eroded.

Sapphire

Colour: blue, blue-violet, yellow, white
Hardness: 9
Composition: Al_2O_3 + Fe & Ti (aluminium oxide)
Qualities: encouraging spiritually aware, regulating
Main chakra: brow, crown

Myth and history

Sapphire has always been one of the most precious of gemstones, both for its colour and its hardness, second only to diamond. India and Sri Lanka both have many famous deposits that have been actively mined for many thousands of years.

It is said that, traditionally, royalty wore sapphires to protect themselves from harm and from the envy of others. The rich blue of the stone was thought to suggest a pure sky that encouraged divine favour and spiritual blessings. Sapphire was also thought to enable seers to better understand the most obscure and difficult of oracles. The stone was used as well to influence all sorts of spirits, and so became a favourite of witches and magicians.

Star sapphire is the most auspicious type of sapphire. The star formation occurs in the transparent stones, where microscopic intergrown crystals reflect the light on the polished dome of

Suggested Crystal Readings

Sapphire in centre/First House
People expect you to be able to see all aspects of the situation.

Sapphire in southeast/Second House
Clarify your motives before taking action.

Sapphire in east/Third House
Put your ideas across clearly, precisely, and with minimal fuss.

Sapphire in north/Fourth House
Make an effort to finish jobs and projects at home.

Sapphire in west/Fifth House
Take up challenges and start developing and honing new skills.

Sapphire in Sixth House
Clarity and precision are needed at work.

Sapphire in southwest/Seventh House
Take yourself and your partner to a peaceful, natural setting.

Sapphire in Eighth House
See if you can put your resources to better use.

Sapphire in northeast/Ninth House
Focus your energy on a few specific areas rather than on broad bands of interest.

Sapphire in south/Tenth House
You have the opportunity to relaunch or expand your role.

Sapphire in northwest/Eleventh House
Be choosy about your social activities – don't commit yourself to too many events.

Sapphire in Twelfth House
If you want to get some peace, you must detach yourself from the emotions of those around you.

Personality

Sapphire represents a very observant person who likes to stand back and watch rather than take part. This person also works with spiritual and psychic energies as a matter of course – not for the glamour of it.

Energy

Expansive, precise, understanding.

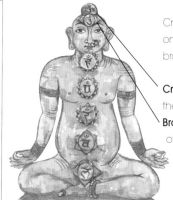

Crystals are placed on the crown and brow chakras.

Crown chakra top of the head
Brow chakra centre of forehead

183

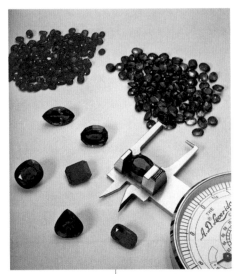

Above Sapphires for the gem industry are valued by their richness of colour and lack of internal flaws.

a cabochon cut in a perfect six-pointed star. The great explorer Sir Richard Burton had a star sapphire with him always – not just for luck, but also as a way to impress others to do his bidding. In medieval Germany, star sapphire was known as the "victory stone," and was considered a powerful protection from the evil eye.

Spiritual and healing properties

Sapphire has a calming and regulating effect on many systems of the body. Wherever there is overactivity and a build-up of tension, sapphire brings a cool relaxation. Anxiety eases, there is a smoother flow of communication and personal expression, and the higher mind is stimulated, enabling an improved experiencing of the subtle states of perception.

Star sapphire emphasises the spiritual energies of the mineral, aiding clairvoyance and visionary experience. All types and colours of sapphire can be useful aids to meditation.

Divinatory interpretation

Sapphire in a cast indicates the need for great precision and clarity in all actions. If emotions are troubled, this stone suggests the need for reestablishing a collected, cool, and considered state. It is important to understand the motivations of those around you, and to be able to properly interpret what people are saying and why.

In areas where problems exist, sapphire shows a relaxed, harmonious, and rejuvenating environment. However, acting from a purely personal viewpoint and in response to one's own emotional states is to be avoided in the areas where sapphire falls in a reading. Keep

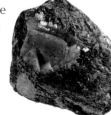

your wits about you and pay attention to clues that may inform you as to the true feelings of the people you are dealing with. In keeping your mind attentive, you may notice, too, how you are reacting to others. You might be surprised at how easy it is for your immediate emotional responses to confuse and muddy the situation.

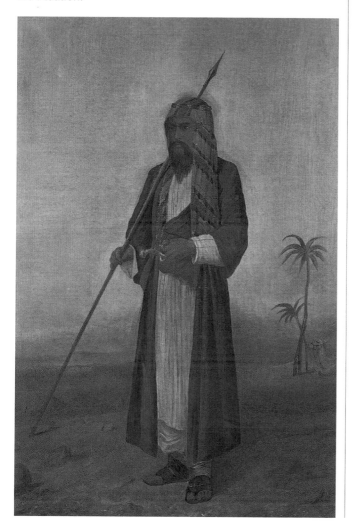

Left Explorer Richard Burton owned a large star sapphire and claimed it brought prompt service wherever he went.

Blue Lace Agate

The delicate and subtle bandings within this crystal make it one of the rarest and most popular of the agates.

Technically, agates are a type of chalcedony quartz, but they are often separately identified because of the distinct bands of microcrystalline layers. Blue lace agate is considered a variety of quartz, albeit an uncommon one.

Agates commonly form when volcanic rocks containing crevices and cavities become filled with quartz solutions as they cool. Each layer of agate crystallizes differently, depending on conditions, temperature, and impurities present, so that agate sizes and colours vary, and a distinctive banding is created. When not completely filled with bands of microcrystals, the centre of an agate can contain clear quartz, amethyst, or smoky quartz crystals.

As agate is harder than the surrounding bedrock, it can often be found in topsoil and on beaches as individual nodules.

Blue lace agate

Colour: bands of blue and white
Hardness: 6.5
Composition: SiO_2 (agate quartz)
Qualities: calming, uplifting
Main chakra: throat

Myth and history

Agate was highly valued by many ancient civilizations, including the Egyptians and Sumerians, even though today it is regarded only as a semiprecious stone. It was named by the Greek scholar Theophrastus in the third century BC after the river Achates, located in present-day Sicily, where it was first discovered. The Greeks became renowned for their skills in carving agate, and some of their most famous artists used the stone, including Pyrgoteles, the engraver of Alexander the Great.

In the Roman Empire, agate was used for all sorts of decorative carving and jewellery, including seal rings, which originally only

Suggested Crystal Readings

Blue lace agate in centre/First House
Be aware of what your body language may be indicating to others.

Blue lace agate in southeast/Second House
Your beliefs about a situation may be impeding your judgment.

Blue lace agate in east/Third House
Be willing to listen to others and to hear what they are saying.

Blue lace agate in north/Fourth House
You really are secure and safe.

Blue lace agate in west/Fifth House
Spend more time in easy conversation and try to enjoy yourself more often.

Blue lace agate in Sixth House
If you feel your health is not as it should be, then do something positive about it.

Blue lace agate in southwest/Seventh House
Be willing to share your thoughts with those who are close to you.

Blue lace agate in Eighth House
Make more of an effort to understand other people's problems.

Blue lace agate in northeast/Ninth House
Make sure you have properly understood the message before you try to pass it on to others.

Blue lace agate in south/Tenth House
Express yourself clearly, to avoid confusion.

Blue lace agate in northwest/Eleventh House
You do not need to believe what everyone else may be saying. Go your own way.

Blue lace agate in Twelfth House
Listen to what your dreams seem to be telling you at the moment.

Personality

This person is perhaps a little vague. He or she is spiritually oriented, and is likely a dreamer as well as a good communicator.

Energy

Communicator, listener.

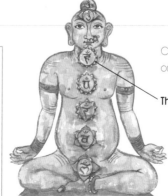

Crystals are placed on the throat chakra.

Throat chakra neck

187

Above This agate cameo displays the profile of Alexander the Great with the rams' horns of the Egyptian god Amun.

Right Agate was a popular stone for carving until modern times. This late eighteenth-century vase was created from a single piece of highly decorative agate.

the upper classes were allowed to own. When it could be cut to show concentric circles, it was valued as a remedy for the evil eye. Even without this particular patterning, agate was thought to strengthen all virtues and provide protection from harm.

Spiritual and healing properties

The blue of this variety of agate is both striking and delicate. The colour strengthens the function of the throat chakra and, like all blue stones, encourages peace, calm, and a sense of quiet detachment. Blue lace agate can be of use wherever there is aggravation or a build-up of energy causing pain, irritation, or inflammation. The energy of blue lace agate is much softer than that of many other blue stones – it tends to be uplifting and supporting, and its subtle variations can suggest the influence of higher spiritual realms.

Divinatory interpretation

Blue lace agate in a reading suggests that many levels of communication are needed, or are going on within the area of the cast. This communication is neither frenetic nor frantic in nature, nor is it necessarily characterised by conflict or argument. The stone's presence simply indicates that there are different ways of understanding and sharing experiences, and that in order to make the most of the situation it is best to acknowledge this fact. This stone also suggests a need be open to communications from unexpected places.

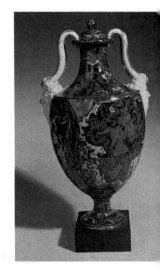

In general, blue lace agate will show an easygoing, light, and enjoyable situation in which communication is important.

Celestite

Celestite is a soft crystal with
a wonderful sky-blue translucence
and powerful energies.

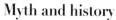

C elestite forms in hydrothermal veins,
as well as in sedimentary and igneous
rock. It usually forms as a result of volcanic
activity, especially near the sea, in tabular or
columnar crystals, often with a rhombohedral cross section. The
most common colouration is a rich, transparent blue.

Myth and history

Celestite, also called celestine, derives its name from the Latin
word *caelestis*, meaning heavenly, referring to the fine blue of
its crystals. In India, it traditionally served a religious function;
priests in Bengal would throw celestite powder
onto fires to produce a vivid crimson flame.
Nowadays, this igniting property – caused by the
element strontium – is widely used industrially
to make flares, fireworks, and tracer bullets. It
is also used in some types of food processing, as
well as in the making of glass and ceramics.

Spiritual and healing properties

Celestite has remarkable relaxing and uplifting
abilities. It can help to relieve feelings of sadness, heaviness, or
desperation. This stone can bring about a calm, joyous state,
where the subtle realms and finer levels of reality seem to be more
easily accessible. All of these qualities make celestite a valuable
stone for meditation and intuitive frames of mind. This crystal
can also help to relieve any imbalances in the area of the throat
chakra, affecting communication, expression, and acceptance.
The crown and brow chakras are also stimulated by this crystal.

Celestite

Colour: sky blue, grey, clear
Hardness: 3–3.5
Composition: $SrSO_4$ (strontium
sulfate)
Qualities: light, meditative,
spacious
Main chakra: throat, brow, crown

189

Suggested Crystal Readings

Celestite in centre/First House
Make a special effort to remain focused on matters around you.

Celestite in southeast/Second House
Avoid making any crucial decisions until you can see the situation more clearly.

Celestite in east/Third House
Unexpected meetings could prove to be very beneficial.

Celestite in north/Fourth House
Make your home a peaceful haven for visitors.

Celestite in west/Fifth House
Romantic encounters and other chance meetings are likely at this time.

Celestite in Sixth House
It may be difficult to focus on practicalities at the moment.

Celestite in southwest/Seventh House
Your dream of a perfect romantic partner is preventing you from seeing what you already have.

Celestite in Eighth House
There will be unexpected alterations to your plans.

Celestite in northeast/Ninth House
Wise words from others should be heeded.

Celestite in south/Tenth House
Your dreams and wishes will help keep you focused on the goal.

Celestite in northwest/Eleventh House
Take time to be with others of similar philosophical backgrounds.

Celestite in Twelfth House
You need to rest and recuperate. Leave the world behind for a while.

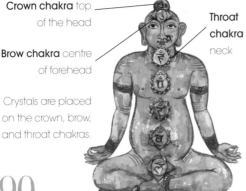

Crown chakra top of the head

Brow chakra centre of forehead

Crystals are placed on the crown, brow, and throat chakras.

Throat chakra neck

Personality

A celestite personality will tend to be in a world of their own: dreamy and contemplative, perhaps a little distant, and completely removed from everyday preoccupations.

Energy

Otherworldly, dreamy, spiritual.

Divinatory interpretation

In a reading, celestite indicates the presence of spiritual influences. These influences may take the form of coincidences, lucky breaks, unexpected meetings, or simply of time spent in a pleasant, dreamy state.

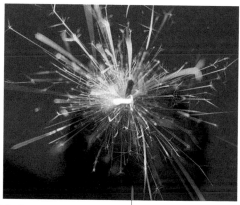

Celestite can suggest the lifting of a heavy mood, the improvement of difficult circumstances, and the ability to see beyond problems. A safe, nurturing space is shown that will help recuperation and will reestablish a balanced calm once more. One must be cautious when this stone appears, however, not to sink too deeply into any otherworldly, dreamy reverie. Heightened states of awareness must always be grounded in everyday reality if they are to be of value.

In a negative placement, celestite might indicate an escape from reality into a fantasy world if other stones nearby show a lack of practical energy.

Left and Below

Fireworks are the combustion of many different materials, each one showing a different brilliant colour. Celestite is typically the source of the deep red displays.

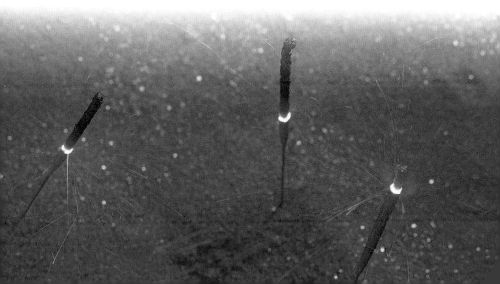

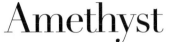

Amethyst

One of the most popular semiprecious stones, amethyst is produced in a variety of transparent purple shades.

Amethyst is a common variety of quartz. It grows in geodes – crystal-filled spherical cavities that are found within volcanic rock. Despite its popularity, amethyst is classed as semiprecious because of the rarity of gem-quality stones. Amethyst tends to have colour zones throughout each crystal rather than consistent shading. Careful heating can disperse the colour more evenly, but too much heat will turn the stone to yellow, brown, or green. Some amethysts will fade in daylight very quickly. The cause of the stone's colouration is not known for certain, but one possibility may be a combination of iron atoms in the lattice and radioactive decay.

Amethyst

Colour: pale violet to deep purple
Hardness: 7
Composition: SiO_2 (quartz)
Qualities: clarifying, calming, integrating
Main chakra: brow, crown

Myth and history

Amethyst has adorned jewellery for at least 5,000 years. It was cut for seals and rings by the ancient Egyptians, and was popular in both classical Greece and Rome.

There was a common belief that amethyst could prevent the worst effects of too much alcohol, and thus derived its name from the Greek word *amethystos*, meaning "not drunken." A classical tale relates that Bacchus, god of wine and ecstasy, accidentally cursed a young maiden, Amethistos, who was on her way to Diana's temple. About to be torn to pieces by wild animals, she prayed to Diana (moon goddess of chastity and the hunt), who turned her into white stone. Bacchus, acknowledging his error, poured wine over the transformed girl, turning the stone to amethyst.

Suggested Crystal Readings

Amethyst in centre/First House
You have a need to appear to others as calm and in control.

Amethyst in southeast/Second House
Tension could build up and create headaches or stomach upsets. Learn to relax.

Amethyst in east/Third House
Be calm and reasonable in your communications.

Amethyst in north/Fourth House
Keep the balance between your work and home life. Don't let either one dominate.

Amethyst in west/Fifth House
Curb any impulse to take risks or to gamble with money or emotions.

Amethyst in Sixth House
Look after your health as a priority now.

Amethyst in southwest/Seventh House
It is time to make peace with anyone who seems antagonistic toward you.

Amethyst in Eighth House
First impressions can be misleading, so be cautious in making any commitments.

Amethyst in northeast/Ninth House
Avoid being overly enthusiastic in any current plans.

Amethyst in south/Tenth House
Figure out what your priorities are and stick with them.

Amethyst in northwest/Eleventh House
Peaceful and relaxing activities will be helpful at this time.

Amethyst in Twelfth House
You may be experiencing sleep difficulties, restlessness, and anxiety at the moment. Try your hardest to relax.

Personality

An amethyst character will be levelheaded, generous, and fair, and may be a religious professional. If their spiritual interests have been repressed, there may be an excessive use of alcohol or narcotics.

Energy

Self-controlled, calm, considerate.

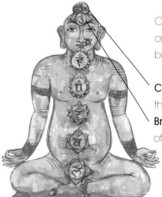

Crystals are placed on the crown and brow chakras.

Crown chakra top of the head
Brow chakra centre of forehead

193

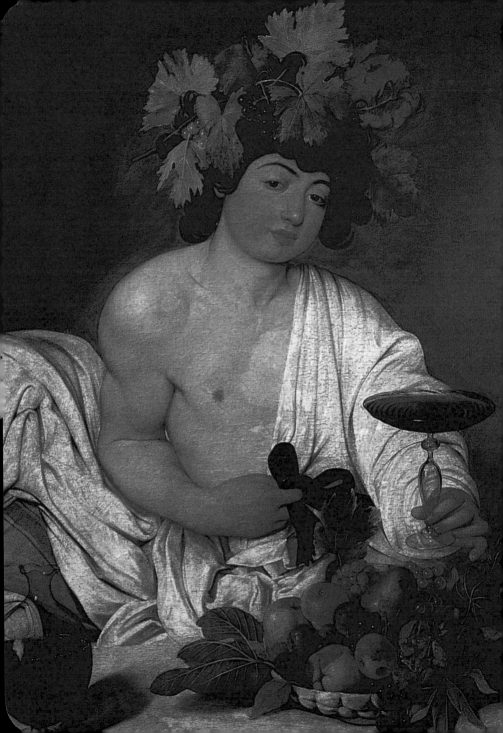

During the Middle Ages, amethyst was generally associated with an upright and sober mentality. It was thought to calm the passions, increase shrewdness and intelligence, and provide protection from enemies, wild animals, and disease.

Spiritual and healing properties

Amethyst is primarily a stone of the mind. It helps to bring calmness and clarity where there is anxiety and confusion. It also integrates and balances all systems of the body, and is thus an important universal healing stone. Amethyst can be a useful stone for meditation and other spiritual exercises, as it calms both the mind and the emotions while keeping awareness sharp and focused. Intuition is also enhanced.

Divinatory interpretation

Amethyst appearing in a reading suggests that there is a need for calm, sober deliberation if decisions are to be made. If the stone falls within areas pertaining to health, there may be issues concerning anxiety, nervous headaches, digestive disorders (often linked to levels of mental stress), or physical coordination problems.

Amethyst in a reading can also be seen as a warning that a degree of self-discipline is needed; now is not the time to have a wild night out on the town. Begin to put things in order, make sense of your priorities, and make sure you are not overdoing anything in your life. Insure that you have your feet on the ground and are not getting carried away by unrealistic, grandiose schemes. Imagination is very important, but it must be focused on practical goals.

Facing Page The ancient Greek god Bacchus symbolized the unruly and unpredictable energies that amethyst is thought to moderate.

Above Amethyst was a fashionable gemstone for Victorian jewellery, as it symbolized sobriety, reliability, and spiritual aspiration.

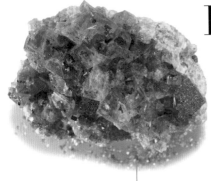

Fluorite

Fluorite is one of the most attractive of all mineral forms, and has a wide range of industrial uses.

Fluorite

Colour: purple, blue, green, yellow, clear

Hardness: 4

Composition: CaF_2 (calcium fluoride)

Qualities: inventive, innovative, coordinated

Main chakra: brow

Right Fluorite not only encourages the invention of new technologies – it can also be a key ingredient within them.

Fluorite is a common mineral that forms when mineral veins come into contact with hot water. It is often found together with such minerals as silver, tin, and lead, and thus miners have been familiar with this mineral for many centuries. Fluorite appears in a wide range of colours. The cubic form of its crystals can result in striking clusters of stepped and pyramidal shapes.

Myth and history

The Romans imported fluorite from Iran (then known as Parthia) to make the famous murrhine vases. The Greeks also used fluorite as an ornamental stone. Because of its value, fluorite was widely imitated using special glass-making processes.

Fluorite takes its name from the Latin word *fluere*, meaning "to flow." It is so named because of its low melting temperature. In some areas of the world, miners called it the "ore flower."

In the early nineteenth century it was discovered that, when certain frequencies of light were shone upon the stone, it would emit light of a different colour. This characteristic became known as "fluorescence."

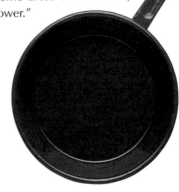

196

Suggested Crystal Readings

Fluorite in centre/First House
Remain clearheaded and cautious.

Fluorite in southeast/Second House
Be completely practical in approaching problem-solving.

Fluorite in east/Third House
Don't go ahead with your plans before consulting others about them.

Fluorite in north/Fourth House
You may find yourself forgetting facts and figures unless you get more rest.

Fluorite in west/Fifth House
Walking, swimming, or yoga will help you think more clearly.

Fluorite in Sixth House
Make plans before you rush into any activity associated with work.

Fluorite in southwest/Seventh House
You need to take into account the needs of other people, and to compromise slightly.

Fluorite in Eighth House
The timing of any financial dealings may be crucial.

Fluorite in northeast/Ninth House
All sides of a situation must be seen in order to understand what is going on.

Fluorite in south/Tenth House
Make sure your planning is thorough.

Fluorite in northwest/Eleventh House
You may be asked to plan and organise joint ventures and activities.

Fluorite in Twelfth House
You need some time alone to clarify your plans.

Personality

Fluorite represents a designer or inventor. These people may seem to be ahead of their time, and typically offer innovative suggestions regarding ways to increase efficiency.

Energy

Inventive, coordinated, integrated.

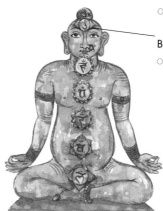

Crystals are placed on the brow chakra.

Brow chakra centre of forehead

197

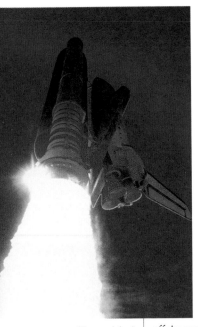

Above Most technological advances involve a moment of inspiration followed by painstaking planning. Fluorite can encourage and help organise the inventive mind.

Today, fluorite is a very important industrial mineral. It is the main source for the fluorine gas and hydrofluoric acid used to make steel, enamel, and glassware, and is also used in refrigerator coolants (chlorofluorocarbons, or CFCs), rocket technology, and nonstick coatings. It is used as a disinfectant as well. Although soft and easily cleavable, fluorite is sometimes used as a gemstone – usually cut as a cabochon or relief carving.

Spiritual and healing properties

Fluorite helps to assimilate ideas and information from many different sources into conscious awareness. Sudden ideas, inventions, new technologies, and dreams of the future are all encouraged by this stone. Working with the brow chakra, fluorite focuses its energy on the functioning of the mind, helping physical coordination, dexterity, balance, and learning skills. Orderliness and an increased structure in one's affairs are encouraged. Fluorite also helps to maintain the integrity of the skeletal system.

Divinatory interpretation

This crystal works at many different levels, and encourages multilevel activity. In a reading, it indicates that now is the time to make detailed plans. It is essential that circumstances be given some firm shape and direction, or present opportunities may melt away.

Fluorite suggests that you need to sit down and think carefully about what you want and how you can practically achieve your goals. Rather than diving straight into action, sit back and allow new ideas to form. Think about how goals can be achieved and then, in a methodical and organised way, begin to move toward them.

In a negative placement, fluorite suggests cloudy thinking, wasted energy on inappropriate activities, clumsiness, and either too much time daydreaming or not enough time thinking about a specific situation.

Sugilite

First identified in Japan in 1944, sugilite is named after its discoverer, Kenichi Sugi.

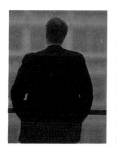

S ugilite forms deep under the ground within volcanic rock. It is part of a group of closely related minerals named osumilites, from the Osumi region of Japan. All osumilites are complex silicates of potassium, sodium, iron, magnesium, and aluminium, and all are very similar in appearance.

Sugilite was not confirmed as a distinct mineral until 1976. It forms as aggregates of small hexagonal crystals, or as massive microcrystalline blocks. The best gem-quality sugilite comes from India and especially South Africa, where it is called royal azel, lavulite, or royal lavulite.

Sugilite

Colour: purple, pink, lilac
Hardness: 5.5–6.5
Composition: $KNa_2 (Fe^{2+} + Mn^2 + Al)_2 Li_3 Si_{12} O_{30}$
Qualities: integrating, balancing
Main chakra: crown

Myth and history

Over two hundred new minerals are identified each year, but few become popular with jewellers or healers. Because of its ability to be easily worked and polished, sugilite is a favourite of jewellers, who cut it into beads and cabochons. Its deep, rich colouring has also made it popular with healers, who believe that it can help integrate spiritual qualities into the modern age.

Spiritual and healing properties

Sugilite works very well at the crown chakra, which acts as a channel for the entrance of universal energies into the body and mind and defines, sustains, and energises the whole chakra system. Sugilite helps the crown to integrate this influx of spiritual energy into daily living. It can be

Above There is often a discrepancy between the lives we lead and the dreams we hold dear. Sugilite can help reintegrate our spiritual integrity into our everyday lives.

199

Suggested Crystal Readings

Sugilite in centre/First House
You may feel a need to be seen living your beliefs instead of toeing the line.

Sugilite in southeast/Second House
Isolating yourself from group activities is not the best action at the moment.

Sugilite in east/Third House
Discussions and debates with friends could be helpful for you at present.

Sugilite in north/Fourth House
You may feel out of step from the rest of your family at the moment.

Sugilite in west/Fifth House
Take time to create an original and useful object.

Sugilite in Sixth House
Both your health and your work may be suffering because of internal tensions concerning a conflict of material and spiritual goals in your life.

Sugilite in southwest/Seventh House
Disagreements can be resolved by looking for common ground.

Sugilite in Eighth House
Avoid schemes that seem to be offering something for nothing.

Sugilite in northeast/Ninth House
Opportunities need to be looked at realistically.

Sugilite in south/Tenth House
Your plans should take into account your ideals as well as practical possibilities.

Sugilite in northwest/Eleventh House
A group you are involved with needs to improve its focus in order to succeed.

Sugilite in Twelfth House
Helping others is a useful way to expand your experience.

Crystals are placed on the crown chakra.

Crown chakra top of the head

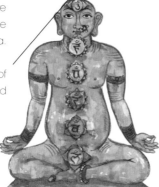

Personality
Sugilite represents a sensitive person with a lively imagination, but this person likely finds it difficult to socialise with others on an everyday basis.

Energy
Integrated, balanced, alienated.

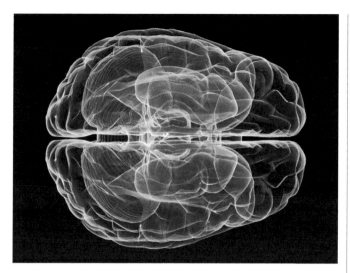

useful for those who are very sensitive, or who find it difficult to feel at ease with modern life.

Sugulite also strengthens all functions of the nervous system. It is particularly helpful where there is a lack of coordination between the left and right hemispheres of the brain, affecting physical coordination.

Divinatory interpretation

In the areas in which it falls, sugilite suggests the need for a greater integration between spiritual and physical qualities. It may be that the questioner's ideals are too rarefied, and that too much is expected from the effort that is being made. On the other hand, the situation may be suffering because spiritual aspects are being ignored in favour of obvious material benefits. If the stone appears in an area relating to health, it may suggest the need to watch out for clumsiness or a lack of dexterity, as this may be the cause of future problems.

Sugilite may also suggest a sense of alienation within one's surroundings, or of being out of step or perhaps out of one's depth. This will likely be an emotional or personal belief rather than a true evaluation of the situation. Look for common themes and shared aspirations instead of differences in approach and apparent faults.

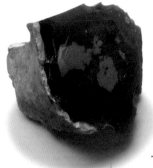

Flint

Flint tools such as arrowheads and axes are among the earliest examples of prehistoric technology.

F lint is a variety of quartz that is created on sea beds when limestone hardens into nodules, or when it is replaced by silica. Because of this origin, it is commonly found together with chalk and the remains of ancient microscopic sea creatures, and may itself contain fossils. Dark grey in colour, flint weathers to a white crust upon exposure to air.

Myth and history

The name for this mineral may derive from the old Swedish word flinta, meaning splinter of stone; or it may come from the Greek word plinthos, meaning brick. Flint is fine-grained and very hard, but when struck sharply, it will defoliate in characteristic conchoidal (shell-shaped) flakes on the face opposite the blow. This defoliation allows nodules of flint to be worked very precisely.

For thousands of years, flint technology was the mainstay of human survival skills.

Because flint sparks when struck, it was used to create fire. Our ancestors also used flint to make first simple and then very sophisticated and effective tools for a wide range of everyday needs. With the advent of gunpowder-based weapons in the sixteenth century, it was used in the firing mechanisms of guns until the mid-nineteenth century. Today, flint is used primarily as a building material in areas where it is commonly found, such as southern England. It is also used in road construction, and as an abrasive.

Flint

Colour: blue-grey, grey, black
Hardness: 7
Composition: SiO_2
Qualities: strengthening, regenerating
Main chakra: solar plexus

Suggested Crystal Readings

Flint in centre/First House
You need to appear strong, but at the same time, open to new ideas.

Flint in southeast/Second House
Have faith in your own strength and resolve.

Flint in east/Third House
Your ideas may seem out of step with those around you, but you are right.

Flint in north/Fourth House
Reassess your resources and assets and create a more secure base.

Flint in west/Fifth House
Be on the lookout for new experiences or hobbies.

Flint in Sixth House
Be willing to give others a helping hand in their quest for a new start.

Flint in southwest/Seventh House
Look to the root of any disagreements before trying to settle differences.

Flint in Eighth House
Unexpected events may seem to create havoc, but will have positive outcomes.

Flint in northeast/Ninth House
Trust your intuition to guide you to the next stage of the current situation.

Flint in south/Tenth House
Dare to be different and to see the present situation through, staying focused on your target.

Flint in northwest/Eleventh House
New friends and a new social scene have their thrills, but they may be tiring you out.

Flint in Twelfth House
You may be restless for no apparent reason. Keeping busy may help.

Personality

Practical and inventive, the flint personality may also appear to be unresponsive and rigid, but with the right stimulus, this personality will help out whenever possible.

Energy

Strong, innovative, resourceful.

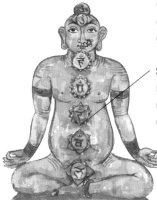

Crystals are placed on the solar plexus chakra.

Solar plexus chakra
midway between navel and base of ribs

Because the shape of a flint nodule resembles bone, in ancient times it naturally became associated with the spirits of the Earth, the fairy folk, and ancestral spirits.

Spiritual and healing properties

Flint helps the body to repair itself at every level, and also helps with the assimilation of nutrients. It has been used in many cultures as protection against negative influences, which it is said to absorb. It is also thought to improve self-confidence, and to help provide a strong sense of connection and belonging in relation to other people and the world in general.

This hard stone strengthens all of the subtle systems of the body, but focuses most at the level of the solar plexus chakra, imbuing confidence, personal power, and assimilation of information on all levels.

Divinatory interpretation

Flint is the stone of invention and innovation. In its natural formation, it is just a lump of rock, but with a bit of work, it can be transformed into a precise tool. In a positive placement, flint shows strength and ingenuity. However, in a difficult position, it may suggest conflict and negative influences. If this is the case, then the positive qualities of flint will help you escape from the aggression you are facing. It is usually within the conflict itself that the resolution can be found. Don't look elsewhere: examine the flashpoints – the sparks that have ignited the trouble – and learn to control them so that they can work to everyone's advantage.   Remember that a fire can burn down a house, but it can also cook a meal. Use your skills to mould the situation constructively.

Above Flint has the property of sparking when struck with steel, and thus it was a common firearm component in the late seventeenth century.

Right Found in many regions of the world, prehistoric flint arrowheads can tell us a great deal about how our ancestors lived and about their level of sophistication.

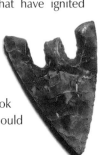
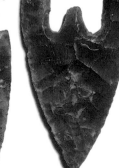

Hematite

Hematite is seen as the sacred blood of the Earth Mother herself, and has been valued for longer than any other mineral.

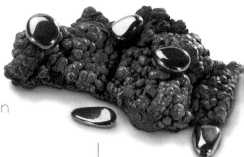

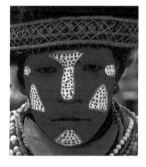

Hematite is a common mineral forming in igneous rock from iron-rich water. Crystals are uncommon; more often, hematite forms kidney-shaped masses. The high iron content of this mineral makes it an important industrial source of iron.

Left The use of red pigment is one of the most ancient methods of denoting the ritually prepared or sanctified individual.

Myth and history

Hundreds of thousands of years before the smelting of iron was discovered, hematite ore was a major trade item. In its metallic form, it was used for jewellery and ornaments, but most precious was the fine-grained ochre – an earthy iron-rich compound used as a sacred red pigment. The oldest mines known are in South Africa, where the hematite was laboriously dug out of open pits with wood and bone picks. These mines were in continuous use for many thousands of years. Once a pit was exhausted, it was carefully refilled to restore the sacred place to its original state.

The graves and bones of Neanderthal man have been found packed in red ochre, suggesting that, even at this early time, man recognised the spiritual symbolism of this life-giving blood of Mother Earth. Hematite continues to be an important source of red pigment today.

Hematite

Colour: metallic silver-grey to brick red
Hardness: 5–6
Composition: Fe_2O_3 (iron oxide)
Qualities: grounding, solidity
Main chakra: base

205

Suggested Crystal Readings

Hematite in centre/First House
You have a need to be seen by others as strong, dependable, and loyal.

Hematite in southeast/Second House
Unwillingness to change a point of view could be clouding issues at the moment.

Hematite in east/Third House
Straight talking is needed to maintain your position, even if you are unsure of the views of others.

Hematite in north/Fourth House
Take time to repair those items in your home that keep it secure.

Hematite in west/Fifth House
You need to put more effort into your leisure time if you wish to actually do the things you keep thinking about.

Hematite in Sixth House
Commit yourself to tackling work with more flexibility.

Hematite in southwest/Seventh House
Secure relationships can become boring. Make sure you are not taking others for granted.

Hematite in Eighth House
Any change in your financial situation should be carefully examined.

Hematite in northeast/Ninth House
Time to consolidate, not expand into new areas. Slow things down!

Hematite in south/Tenth House
Your ability to integrate your skills has helped you to get what you want.

Hematite in northwest/Eleventh House
Don't try to deceive your friends – they know you too well. Just be you.

Hematite in Twelfth House
Look beyond the obvious to find the strength and security you need.

Crystals are placed on the base chakra.

Base (root) chakra
base of spine
(perineum)

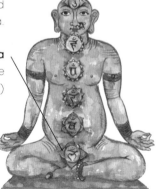

Personality

This crystal represents someone who is solid and dependable. They may appear boring, but he or she has a strengthening and stabilising effect. He or she may have spiritual experiences, but will keep this a secret.

Energy

Strong, secure, straightforward

Spiritual and healing properties

With its iron content, hematite has a strengthening influence on the physical body – especially the blood, body temperature, and circulatory system. Of all the grounding stones, hematite is perhaps the surest – very few people fail to be brought down to a steady, focused state due to its stabilizing influence on the physical body.

Traditionally, iron was held to be the only protection against the Faerie Kingdoms, and today, hematite will prevent you from being taken "away with the fairies" or, to use another colloquialism for an unfocused mind, being "spaced out."

When used by a fully

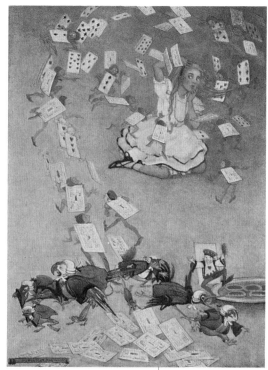

balanced personality, hematite can provide access to spirit travel and astral worlds.

Divinatory interpretation

Iron is a strong but brittle metal, and these characteristics provide a clue to its divinatory meanings. Hematite appearing in a cast will show solid foundations upon which to build. In a positive placement, it will encourage the solidification of other energies close to it. In this way, hematite can crystallise a situation so that it becomes clear and visible to all. In a negative placement, hematite can indicate stubbornness, inflexibility, or an inability to move away from a current condition.

Hematite appears to be a shiny silver metal, but when powdered, it becomes red. This transformation shows us that it is sometimes necessary to look beyond the surface of matters.

Above Fairy tales and folk legends instruct us on the attractions and pitfalls of entering the spirit world unprepared. In this realm, iron is one of the main protections against harm.

207

Schorl (black tourmaline)

Schorl brings the strength and stability of the planet Earth into the human aura.

Tourmaline is formed deep in fractures of the Earth's crust, along with minerals such as quartz, mica, and feldspar. It forms long, thin, three-sided crystals with parallel striations along the length of the prism. Schorl, the black variety, is the most common. Tourmaline is unusual in that, when it is heated, one end of the crystal becomes charged electrically positive, while the other end has a negative charge. This makes it useful as a switching device in many types of machinery.

Schorl

Colour: black, opaque, or slightly translucent

Hardness: 7.5

Composition: Na $(Mg,Fe,Li,Mn,Al)_3 Al_6(BO_3) Si6 O_{18} (OHF)_4$ (complex borosilicate)

Qualities: protective, structuring, grounding

Main chakra: base

Facing Page Schorl can help realign the structural aspects of the body, such as the bones and the muscles. Pulls and strains are often eased with the help of this crystal.

Myth and history

The Ancient Greeks and Romans are known to have turned the coloured varieties of tourmaline into magical gemstones. During the Middle Ages, tourmaline was not identified as a distinct mineral, as it so closely resembled the colour of other gemstones. Later, Dutch traders visiting Ceylon (present-day Sri Lanka) came across tourmaline, then called turmali (meaning many-coloured), and introduced it as a gemstone into eighteenth-century Europe.

Spiritual and healing properties

Schorl is one of the best stones to use for protection from all sorts of negativity. The stone will deflect, rather than absorb, energy that is unbalancing, creating a safe, neutral space around itself.

This crystal can also bring consciousness back into the physical body very rapidly. It is deeply grounding, and can be used to restore normal awareness after healing or spiritual practices.

Suggested Crystal Readings

Schorl in centre/First House
You have a need to be seen by others as practical and reliable.

Schorl in southeast/Second House
Be careful with your money. Don't purchase unnecessary items.

Schorl in east/Third House
Any communications need to be in harmony with those around you.

Schorl in north/Fourth House
Remember that your roots and home are your foundation. Begin from there.

Schorl in west/Fifth House
Focus your creative skills a little more. This placement is ideal for a new romance.

Schorl in Sixth House
Take extra care with your back when lifting or moving things.

Schorl in southwest/Seventh House
Keep the peace with those you love.

Schorl in Eighth House
Arguments with others may have upset you more than you thought.

Schorl in northeast/Ninth House
Keep your feet firmly on the ground when opportunities come your way.

Schorl in south/Tenth House
Time to consolidate your plans for the future in practical and realistic ways.

Schorl in northwest/Eleventh House
Make time to take walks in natural surroundings with appreciative friends.

Schorl in Twelfth House
Don't allow yourself to get carried away with impractical ideas or vague dreams.

One of schorl's main features is that it is a stone of alignment; it will help the body to make physical readjustments if the bones and muscles are out of place due to injury or strain. It can also align the human body to the energies of planet Earth itself. This makes it a useful stone to carry when travelling around the world or moving somewhere new, as it helps to harmonise personal with planetary energy and reduces the effects of jet lag.

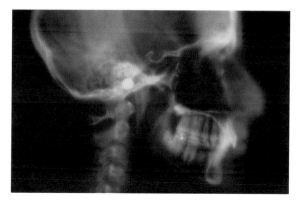

Personality

Black tourmaline can represent people who are down-to-earth, practical, and at home wherever they are. These people may thrive in and seek out unusual or dangerous situations..

Energy

Protective, balancing.

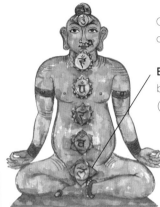

Crystals are placed on the base chakra.

Base (root) chakra
base of spine
(perineum)

Divinatory interpretation

Schorl indicates a need to be in harmony with your surroundings. Without harmony, there may be some danger of encountering negativity on some level – or of simply being clumsy. Either can be avoided by making sure you are fully grounded, focused, and practical in your outlook.

This crystal suggests that the structure of things – the hidden foundations – need to be taken into account. Make sure that the basis of all your actions and relationships is secure and firm.

Right The Earth's energy field varies from place to place. Schorl helps us adjust to these changes when we are travelling.

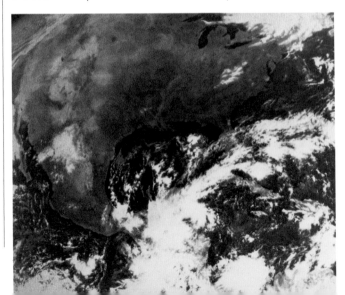

Obsidian

Obsidian is found only in volcanic areas, where it forms from rapidly cooled lava. Born from the fire within the heart of the planet, obsidian can bring a strong sense of determination to conquer fear and face reality in a practical, grounded, and courageous way.

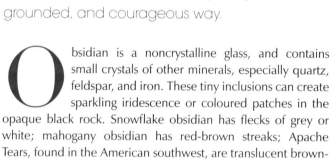

Obsidian is a noncrystalline glass, and contains small crystals of other minerals, especially quartz, feldspar, and iron. These tiny inclusions can create sparkling iridescence or coloured patches in the opaque black rock. Snowflake obsidian has flecks of grey or white; mahogany obsidian has red-brown streaks; Apache Tears, found in the American southwest, are translucent brown-black pebbles of obsidian. Unpolished obsidian should always be handled with caution, as its edges can be very sharp.

Myth and history

Obsidian has been used to make razor-sharp arrowheads and knives since the Stone Age. In Central America, where there is a plentiful supply of obsidian, the Aztecs fashioned clubs, axes, and swords from the stone. It was also used in religious carvings and ornamental regalia.

In Europe during the Middle Ages, obsidian was a popular material with which to make spheres and magical mirrors for scrying (the art of seeing into the future or into other worlds). One well-known scryer was Dr. John Dee, adviser to Queen Elizabeth I of England, Royal Astrologer, diplomat, spy, and occultist. He used an obsidian scrying mirror to communicate

Obsidian

Colour: black with white, grey, or red markings

Hardness: 6

Composition: glass (mix of silicates)

Qualities: grounding, purging, revealing

Main chakra: base

211

Suggested Crystal Readings

Obsidian in centre/First House
Examine how you appear to others. Consider making changes in your appearance or your style of dress.

Obsidian in southeast/Second House
Reassess deeply held beliefs about money before you can move forward.

Obsidian in east/Third House
Think before you speak. If you have strong opinions, wait a while and reconsider.

Obsidian in north/Fourth House
Long-standing difficulties with your family need to be resolved once and for all.

Obsidian in west/Fifth House
The true power of your creative skills is not yet apparent. Examine what is stopping you from fully expressing yourself.

Obsidian in Sixth House
Try not to underestimate the courage it takes to make changes in the way you work.

Obsidian in southwest/Seventh House
Address the painful topics that you have been avoiding with partners.

Obsidian in Eighth House
Financial dealings must be approached with total honesty and openness.

Obsidian in northeast/Ninth House
Look for books or courses that will help you to unlock any talents.

Obsidian in south/Tenth House
Reluctance to alter an aspect of your career may lose you status in the eyes of those who you are trying to impress.

Obsidian in northwest/Eleventh House
Look for possible hidden jealousy from acquaintances. It could upset your current plans – unless dealt with carefully.

Obsidian in Twelfth House
Look to your dreams and daydreams for guidance in your daily life. They will confirm that you already know what you require and what needs to be done.

Crystals are placed on the base chakra.

Base (root) chakra
base of spine
(perineum)

Personality

The typical obsidian person is emotionally volatile and secretive, and is very good at uncovering hidden objects and information.

Energy

Transmuting, deep, hidden.

212

with spirits and, working together with his assistant, Edward Kelley, he developed a system called "Enochian magic," which explores a multitude of spiritual realms ruled over by angelic beings.

Spiritual and healing properties

As a stone that emerges with dramatic force from the depths of the Earth, obsidian is believed by many to bring hidden emotions to the surface. This makes it extremely useful in releasing long-held stresses and buried traumas. Like a volcanic eruption, this process may be a turbulent, unpleasant experience while it is going on, bringing old wounds, fears, and anxieties to the surface before they are released. Transformation always brings change, and change can sometimes be difficult to accept. Nevertheless, change is essential if we are to grow. Obsidian will release only outdated, unwanted remnants of our lives so that we can move forward, unencumbered by the past.

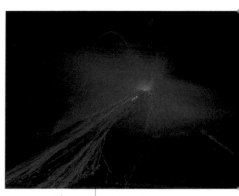

Above Powerful forces can be either constructive or destructive. If they are ignored or not taken into consideration, problems are much more likely to arise.

Divinatory interpretation

Obsidian has a clear relationship with Pluto, both the planetary body and the classical Greek god after which the planet was named. Pluto is the god of the underworld, keeper of hidden treasures.

Whenever obsidian appears in a reading, it is important to look for hidden factors that may be affecting your situation. Unexpected turns of events may be experienced, and any change will be neither slow nor easy. Fear may also be an issue that needs to be dealt with – either your own or other people's. Remember that fear usually arises when there is a feeling that events are beyond our control, or when we cannot see the whole picture. Fear can also appear when you are face to face with something that seems to be more powerful than you.

The nature of obsidian is both fiery and grounding. These qualities will see you through any obsidian-like eruptions, creating a conviction in your own fiery strength and an ability to stand equal to anyone on the planet.

213

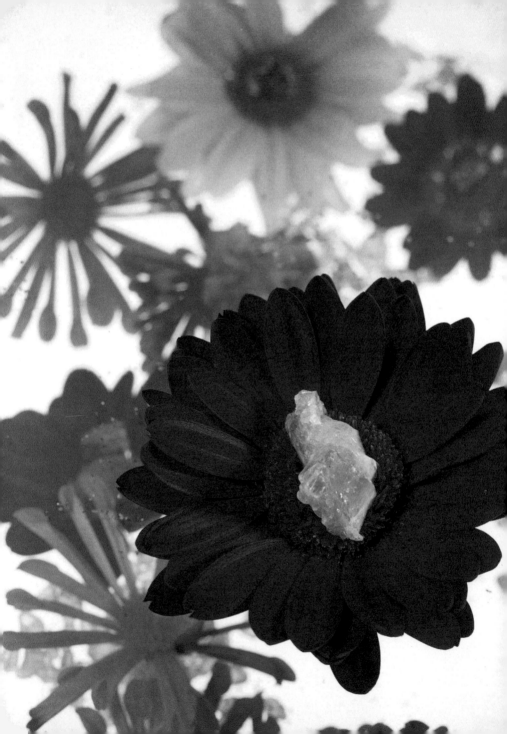

Crystal Magic

Magic is often the next natural step following divination. With divination, we diagnose; with magic, we offer the appropriate medicine. Indeed, like medicine, magic is a powerful tool, and, like the wrong medicine, the wrong magic can do more harm than good. On the following pages are three magical spells involving crystals that can help you improve certain areas of your life.

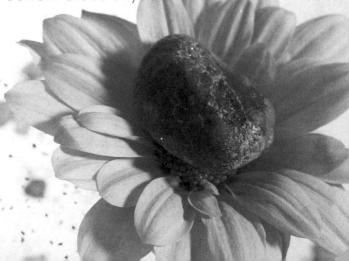

Invisibility and Protection from Harm

This spell can protect you from those people and things that might bear you malice. It should be used only in situations where invisibility will be beneficial, and not in cases where it would be harmful – when crossing the road for example!

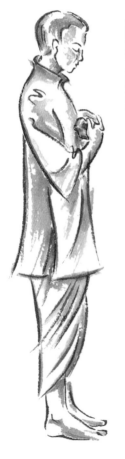

You will need:

- A transparent, clear crystal such as quartz, calcite, or fluorite
- One red stone, one blue stone, one green stone, and one yellow stone
- A bowl or jar of water (a vessel with a dark interior will work best)

Place the bowl of water on a table. Pick up the red stone (representing the element of fire) and say:

> *Stone of fire*
> *to ashes turn all*
> *harm that hunts me.*

Repeat this verse several times while holding the stone to your solar plexus, which is your own fire energy centre.

Put the stone down beside the bowl and say:
> *Hide me from hurt.*

Next, pick up the blue stone (representing the element of water) and say:

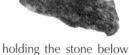

> *Stone of water*
> *melt, dissolve, disperse*
> *all ill that stalks me.*

Repeat this verse several times while holding the stone below your navel, which is your own water centre.

Lay the stone at the opposite side of the bowl to the fire stone and say:
Hide me from hurt.

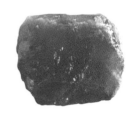

Now pick up the green stone (representing the element of air) and say:
Stone of air
scatter like leaves
ill thoughts and intentions.

Repeat this verse several times while holding the stone to the heart centre in the middle of the chest.
Lay the stone to the left of the fire stone by the bowl and say:
Hide me from hurt.

Pick up the yellow stone (representing the element of earth) and say:
Stone of earth
hold fast and hide
No foes will find me..

Repeat this verse several times while holding the stone at the base of your spine.
Place the stone by the bowl opposite the green stone and say:
Hide me from hurt.

Now, take the clear crystal in your hands and say:
As fire I cannot be held
As air I cannot be seen
As water I flow around all obstacles
As earth I am unshakable

Look at the clear stone and repeat the words "as clear as crystal" many times, while imagining that your whole being has taken on the same transparency as the stone. When this image is clear, carefully place the stone in the bowl. Watch as its edges become indistinct. Occasionally repeat the words "as clear as crystal." To end the spell, thank each element and dismantle the arrangement.

Abundance and Fulfilment

Although it often seems to be linked to external factors, abundance is created internally and at subtle levels of thought and feeling. Dissatisfaction, emptiness, and a sense of poverty are indications that we have become separated and isolated from the beneficial energies of the universe.

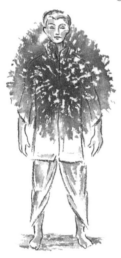

Above Intense concentration is not necessary, especially when the outcome is strongly desired.

You will need:
• One red stone
• A few yellow stones
•A few green stones

First, cleanse the stones you are going to use (see page 36). Begin the spell by sitting quietly and thinking clearly about the reasons why you wish to work the spell. Close your eyes and imagine red roots extending down from where you are in contact with the ground. Feel those energies diving deep toward the centre of the Earth. Send your breath down these roots and feel solid and well rooted.

Now say the words "I am supported." Take the red stone and place it centrally within the space where you are performing the spell. Again, say the words "I am supported."

Close your eyes once again. Visualize golden rays, beams, or threads shooting out from your solar plexus. See them streaming away from you in all directions, contacting everything around, above, and below you. Feel yourself at the centre of a web of golden light. When the image is strong, say "I am nourished."

Take the yellow stones and arrange them concentrically around the red stone. When all the stones are placed, say once again "I am nourished."

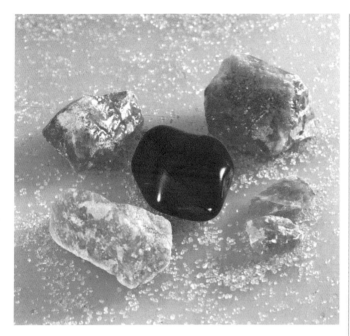

Left Choose stones that you find particularly attractive for your spells. Buying stones for a special purpose will infuse them with the energy of your intention.

Below Visualization does not need microscopic clarity to be effective. Feel the power of the words and let the pictures develop in their own way, at their own speed. Practice will eventually bring clear imagery.

Now close your eyes once more. From the area of light at your solar plexus, imagine a seedling sprouting up toward your heart. As it reaches your heart it forms a large green flower bud. As you watch, the bud slowly opens its beautiful green petals. Green light fills the whole of your body and gently radiates into the space around you. Say, "I am abundant. The wishes in my heart are instantly fulfilled." As you say this, the final petals open up to reveal a brilliant green gemstone or crystal in the heart of the flower. If you have a particular wish, focus your attention on the jewel and think about it.

When you are ready, open your eyes and place the green stones in a concentric circle around the other stones. Again, say "I am abundant. The wishes in my heart are instantly fulfilled."

Sit and look at the stones for a little while. You can now either leave them in place, or clap your hands and clear the stones away. Remembering the jewel within the flower during the day will maintain your energy link.

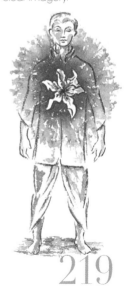

219

Healing Spell

All illness, whether it be physical, emotional, or mental, arises from the wrong sort of energy being in the wrong place at the wrong time. Problems begin when the individual is unable to rebalance his or her energy equilibrium. This spell is designed to lift out excess energy and to return it to a place where it can be used in a life-giving way. Remember that, whatever anyone else may do or wish to do, the healing ultimately comes from the ill person themselves – only the body can repair itself. Sometimes, for various reasons, a person holds onto a diseased state, or continually invites repeating patterns of illness. Only an internal change of heart and mind will end this cycle.

Though you may be successful in removing the subtle levels of imbalance, it is important to realize that the physical body can still take a long time to heal itself. It should also be acknowledged that positive thoughts can be as powerful as anything else. Lastly, remember that it is unwise to become overly attached to outcomes and results. Do your work, and then let the universe do its work.

If you are using the healing spell on someone else, make sure that you have their permission before you start.

You will need:
• A small mirror or a piece of paper with a body outline drawn onto it
•The name or signature and a piece of hair or other item belonging to the person you wish to heal
• A selection of crystals
• A candle
• Incense
• A bowl of water
• A handful of pure rock salt or sea salt

First, create a space that represents the person you wish to help. If you have a small mirror, use this to represent the person. Alternatively, on a good-sized piece of paper, draw a rough outline of a figure or a simple elongated oval shape. This drawing will represent the person – both his or her physical form and his or her surrounding auric field.

Below Although you may be concerned about the health of the person on whose behalf you are performing the spell, it is important that your mind be quiet and that you feel confident that whatever you achieve will be useful.

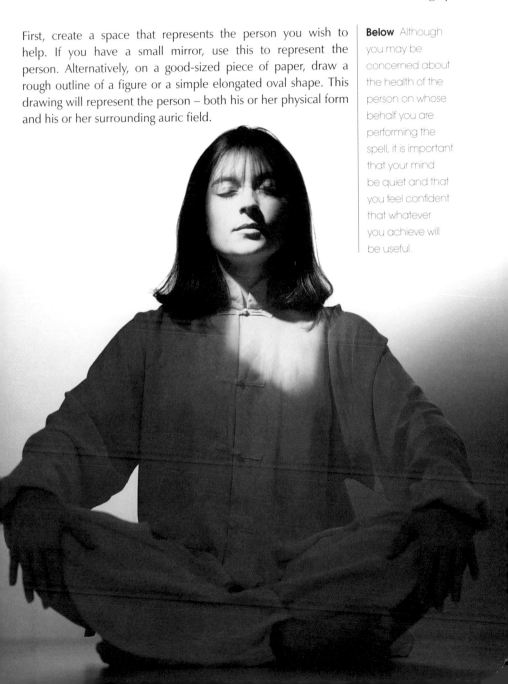

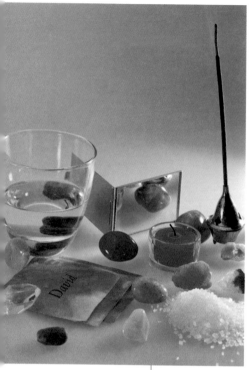

If you have some hair, or a signature or photograph belonging to the person to be healed, place it on your representation and write the person's name underneath it. Take a minute to look at the representation and think about the person and his or her situation.

Next, carefully lay out your crystals and say:
You stones that are the bones
of all things
in all places
through all time;
you stones that help
and heal
come here to me;
you healing spirits
listen to my heart,
show me those that
can help [name of person].

Close your eyes for a moment. When you feel ready, open them and gaze at your stones. Some stones will immediately draw your attention. Pick four of them out and set them aside. Thank the remaining stones and then clear them away.

Sitting down, imagine yourself completely surrounded by an electric-blue aura, especially your hands and fingers. Take each selected stone and, with awareness, slowly pass it over the person's representation, visualizing at the same time imbalances and illness being drawn into the crystal. If you wish to use words here to help you, just say whatever comes to mind.

You may find that certain areas of the representation feel different. Spend more time holding the stone over these areas, letting your intuition guide you. After you have swept over the entire representation, the imbalances within the stone will need to be returned to their proper place in the universe. There are

Above Collect all of the necessary ingredients for the spell together and arrange them in a satisfying way, so that they are within easy reach.

four ways to do this: through fire, air, water, and earth. All four ways are effective for all stones; the choice of which to use for each stone is up to you.

Through fire: Pass the stone above a candle flame and say:
Spirit of Fire
Spirit of Flame
Restore all to light
Restore all to balance

Through water: Sweep the stone through the bowl of water and say:
Spirit of Water
Ocean of cleansing
Wash away all debris
Wash away all dust

Through air: Pass the crystal through incense smoke and say:
Spirit of Air
Breath of life
Bring purity
Bring joy

Through earth: Cover the stone with dry sea or rock salt and say:
Spirit of Earth
Ground of bearing
Return to strength
Return to contentment

After having gone through a cleansing, each stone will be free of any imbalances picked up during the healing process. Where the person is extremely unwell, you can perform the spell four times with each stone, cleansing the stones after each turn.

Throw away the salt and water and extinguish the candle and incense, thanking each element in turn for its help. Wash the stones in cool water. Visualize the blue aura around you and see it expand outward and disperse. Repeat this spell every few days, if necessary.

Index

Page numbers in **bold** refer to illustrations, page numbers in *italic* refer to chakra placement diagrams

abalone shell 16, 79–81, *80*
Abundance and Fulfillment spell 218–19
agate 186, **188**
aggression 85
alabaster **68**
amazonite 160–2, **160**, *161*, **162**
amber 116–19, **116**, **117**, *118*, **119**
amethyst 192–5, **192**, *193*, **194**, **195**
amulets 16, 102–3, 104, 109, 153
anxiety 99, 111, 117, 148, 152, 184, 195
aquamarine 163–5, **163**, *164*, **165**
arthritis 108, **135**
Astrological board 43–5, **43**, **45**, 52, 58–9, **58**
aventurine 150–2, **150**, *151*, **152**
azurite 178–81, **178**, *179*, **180**, **181**

birthstones 32, **32**, **33**
blood 111, 207
bloodstone 136–8, **136**, *137*, **138**
blue lace agate 186–8, **186**, *187*, **188**
Book of Revelation 96, **98**
Book of the Dead, the 102, **104**
brain, the 117, 127, 162, 201, **201**

calcium levels **135**
calmness 64, 72, 86, 132, **150**, 152, 160, 184, 189, 195
carnelian 16, 102–5, **102**, *103*, **104**, **105**
casting techniques 23, 24, 50–1, **51**
celestite 189–91, **189**, *190*, **191**
chakra centres 17, 71
chalcopyrite 133
characteristics 12
circulatory system 135, 138, 158, 207
citrine **11**, 120–2, **120**, *121*, **122–3**
cleansing methods 36, **36**, 223
colour 12–13, 15, 34, 163, **163**
colour therapy 17
Compass board, the 40–3, **41**, **42**, 52, 54–6, **55**
confidence 99, 122, 126, 152, 204
copper 106–8, **106**, *107*, **108**, 133, 178
coral 16
crystal energy 14–15, **14**, **15**
crystal groupings 52, **53**
crystal skulls 62, **64**
crystallisation 10–11

depression 111, 117
detoxification 158
diamond 11
digestive problems 72, 74, 111, 122
divination 21, 22–5, **22**, **23**, **24**, **25**
  ancient methods 22–3
  the Astrological board 43–5, **43**, **45**, 52, 57–9, **58**
  casting **23**, 24, 50–1, **51**
  the Compass board 40–3, **41**, **42**, 52, 54–6, **55**
  crystal reading 26–8
  interpretation 27, 52, **53**, 54–6, 57–9
  pendulum dowsing 48–9, **48**
  preparations 36–9, **36**, **37**, **39**
  scrying 46–7, **47**, 211, 213
diviners 28, 38–9, **39**
dreams 23

emerald 146–9, **146**, *147*, **148**, **149**
emotions, stabilising 81, 85, 86, 99, **101**, 125, 155
energy state, exploring 18
evil eye, the 153, 155, **155**, 188
eyesight 152

far memory 162
fear 132, 148, 152
feldspars 72, 160
feminine energy 74
flint 202–4, **202**, *203*, **204**
fluid balance 74
fluorite 196–8, **196**, *197*, **198**
formation 12, **13**, 14

garnet 88–90, **88**, **89**, *90*, **91**
gemstones 11
geomancy 24
grounding 38–9, 47, 114, 120, 122, 132, 207, 208
gypsum 66, **68**

hawk's eye 112
healing powers 16–17, **17**
Healing spell 220–3, **221**, **222**
heart, the 82, 85, 94, 99, 138, 144, 149, 152, 160
hematite **11**, 205–7, **205**, *206*
human body, the 30, **30**, **31**, 209, **209**

immune system 81, 165, 169, 172
inflammation **106**, 108, 153, 188
inner mind, the 27
Invisibility and Protection from Harm spell 216–17
iron 207, **207**

jade 142–5, **142**, *143*, **144**, **145**
jasper, red 96–8, **96**, *97*, **98**
jewellery **95**, **120**, 127, **145**, **146**, **168**, **169**, **172**, 186, 192, **195**, 199
Jung, Carl 26, **27**

labradorite 69–71, **69**, *70*, **71**
lapis lazuli 170, 174–6, **174**, *175*, **176**, **177**
lepidolite **85–7**, **86**, **87**
light, behavior of 13, 15
lungs 158
lymphatic system 158, 172

magma 10, 12, **13**
malachite 153–5, **153**, *154*, **155**
megalithic sites 76, **78**
milky quartz 76–8, **76**, *77*, **78**
mind, the **29**, 64, 76, **130**, 195, 198
Mo 22
moldavite 139–41, **139**, *140*, **141**
moon, the **74–5**, *75*
moonstone 72–5, **72**, *73*, **74–5**
moss agate 156–9, **156**, *157*, **158**, **159**
mother-of-pearl 81

negativity 66, 135, 152, 169, 208
nervous system 117, 122, 127, 135, 160, 162, 201

obsidian 16, 211–13, **211**, *212*, **213**

pain **106**, 108, 152, 188
peacock ore 133–5, **133**, *134*, **135**

pearls 79–81, **79**, **80**, *80*, **81**
pegmatite 12
pendulum dowsing 48, 49
personal stone, choosing 30, 32, 33
  birthstones 32, **32**, **33**
  preference 33, **34**
  random 35
  stones qualities 34–5
poison 96, **98**
polarity shifts 69, **71**
problem solving 78
pyrite 109–11, **109**, *110*, **111**

quartz 12, 14, **14**, 16, 76. *see also* rock crystal
questioner, the 28

Ragiel's Book of Wings 88
relaxation 81
reproductive ailments 72, 74
resonance, principle of 15
rheumatism 108
rhodonite 99–101, **99**, *100*, **101**
rituals 16
rock crystal 62–5, **62**, *63*, **64**, **65**. *see also* quartz
romance **101**
rose quartz 12, 82–4, **82**, *83*, **84**
rubellite in lepidolite **11**, 85–7, **85**, **86**, **87**, *87*
ruby 11, 92–5, **92**, *93*, **94**
rutilated quartz 127–9, **127**, *128*, **129**

sapphire 182–5, **182**, *183*, **184**, **185**
schorl 208–10, **208**, **209**, **210**, *210*
scrying 24, 46–7, **47**, 211, 213
selenite 66–8, **66**, *67*, **68**
self-worth 82, 122
sensitivity, developing 18–19
shock 104
skeletal system 198
smoky quartz 130–2, **130**, *131*, **132**
snake bites 96, **98**
sodalite 170–2, **170**, *171*, **172**, **173**
spirit travel 207, **207**
spirits 26, **26**
  communication with **17**, **22**, 23
stone circles **40**
stones
  choice for magic **219**
  exploring 18–19
  placing 17, **17**
stress 72, 82, 86, 104, **105**, 120, 159, 181, 213
sugilite 199, 199–201, **200**, **201**

tektites 139, **141**
tiger's eye 112–14, **112**, *113*, **114**, **115**
time 23–4, **24**, **25**
topaz 124–6, **124**, **125**, **126**, *126*
tourmaline 208
turquoise 16, 166–9, **166**, *167*, **168**, **169**

unconscious, the 26–7
universal web theory 26

visualisation **219**

wounds, repair 127

zodiac signs **30**, **31**, 32, **32**